3rd Edition Practical English Conversation for Nurses

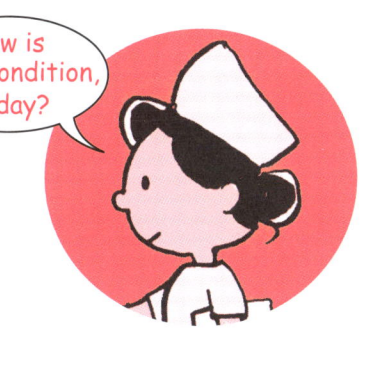

看護英会話入門　　　　第3版

植木　武【共立女子学園名誉教授】／ドレール・トウン　　　　医学書院

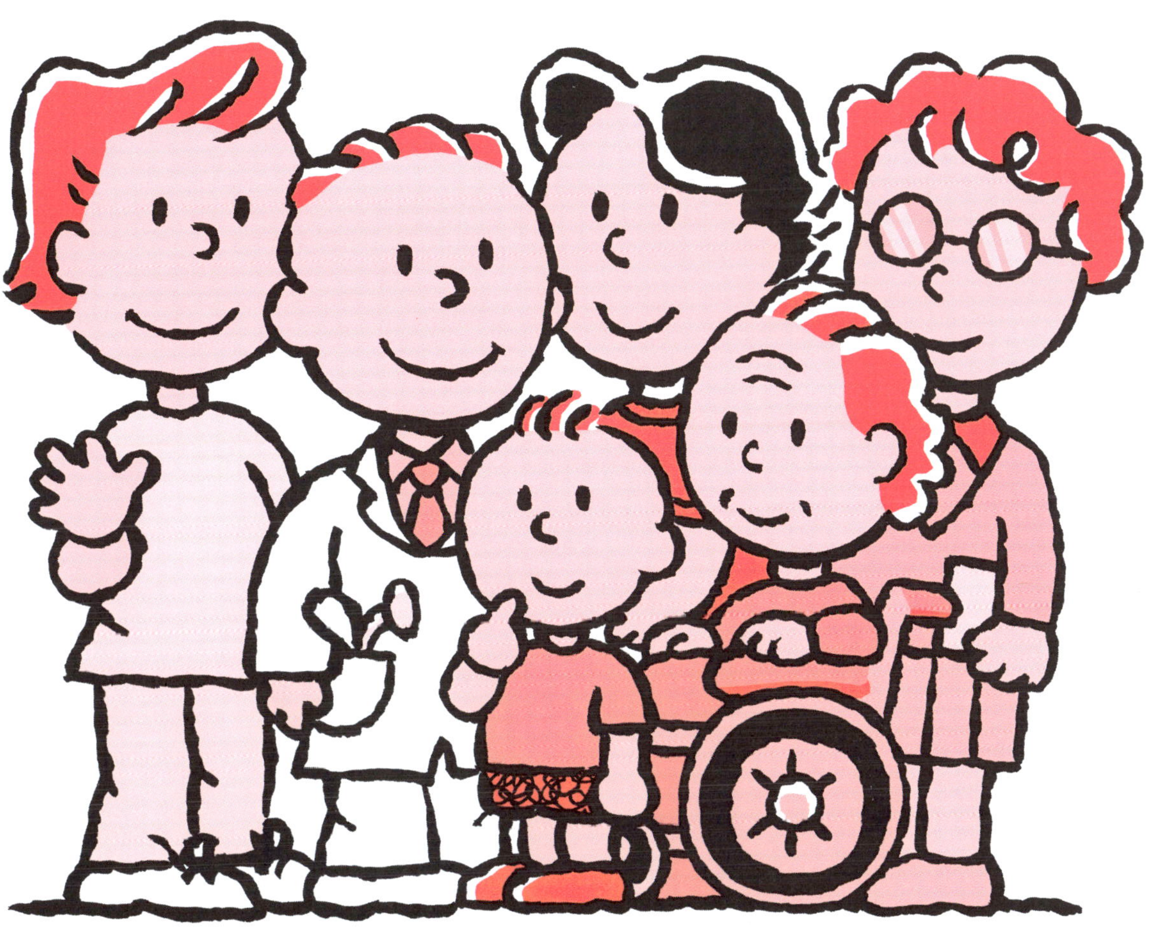

植木　武（Takeshi Ueki）

ブラウン大学人類学部博士課程修了．人類学博士(Ph. D. 1984)．現在，共立女子学園名誉教授．主な著書に『太平洋(共訳)』(法政大学出版局 1989)，『国家の形成』(三一書房 1996)，『コンピュータ英会話入門』(COTE 2000)，『国際理解教育のABC』(東洋出版社 2002)，『国際社会で活躍した日本人』(弘文堂 2009)あり．

ドレール・トウン（Dorelle Toan）

ノース・カロライナ大学看護学部卒業(B. S.)．看護師(R. N.)．サイマル・インターナショナル勤務ののち，医学論文翻訳家として活躍．

Technical Advisor；Juria A. Nale, R.N., B.S.

看護英会話入門　第3版
発　行　1981年 5 月 1 日　　第 1 版第 1 刷
　　　　1991年 3 月15日　　第 1 版第11刷
　　　　1991年 9 月15日　　新訂版第 1 刷
　　　　2003年 3 月 1 日　　新訂版第14刷
　　　　2004年 4 月 1 日　　第 3 版第 1 刷ⓒ
　　　　2022年11月 1 日　　第 3 版第19刷
著　者　植木　武　ドレール・トウン
発行者　株式会社　医学書院
　　　　代表取締役　金原　俊
　　　　〒113-8719　東京都文京区本郷 1-28-23
　　　　電話　03-3817-5600(社内案内)
印刷・製本　真興社

本書の複製権・翻訳権・上映権・譲渡権・貸与権・公衆送信権(送信可能化権を含む)は株式会社医学書院が保有します．

ISBN978-4-260-33327-6

本書を無断で複製する行為(複写，スキャン，デジタルデータ化など)は，「私的使用のための複製」など著作権法上の限られた例外を除き禁じられています．大学，病院，診療所，企業などにおいて，業務上使用する目的(診療，研究活動を含む)で上記の行為を行うことは，その使用範囲が内部的であっても，私的使用には該当せず，違法です．また私的使用に該当する場合であっても，代行業者等の第三者に依頼して上記の行為を行うことは違法となります．

JCOPY〈出版者著作権管理機構　委託出版物〉
本書の無断複製は著作権法上での例外を除き禁じられています．複製される場合は，そのつど事前に，出版者著作権管理機構(電話 03-5244-5088，FAX 03-5244-5089，info@jcopy.or.jp)の許諾を得てください．

序——本書の特徴と使用法

20年にわたって英会話テキストとして使用された『看護英会話入門』を、このたびは全面改訂ということで、より一層臨場感に溢れる会話を取り入れることにした。前書と同じく、外来と病室というシチュエーションで、病院のそれぞれの科で、日常に最も一般的に使用される会話を、看護師(医師、専門技師、歯科衛生師等)を中心に取り上げてみた。ただ、最近では介護施設で活躍する看護師も増加してきたので、介護に関するレッスンも追加した。

以下は本書の特徴である。
1. 各課(L.1～L.25)をAとBに分け、左ページのダイアローグは、必ずしもというわけではないが、基本的にAは少し易しく、Bは少し難しくした。
2. 医学専門用語を中心に、アメリカ標準語発音のルビを加えた。
3. 右ページには、各科において、現場で役に立つ表現や文章も掲示した。
4. 各科(内科、外科等)で頻繁に使用される専門用語を、「Vocabularyをふやそう」として並べた。
5. columnに、病気や海外病院事情などの、知っていると得になる面白い情報を記載した。

次に、本書の使用法を述べることにする。

●個人学習(自習)の場合…(50分)
1. 自分が学習する各レッスンの、A(やや易しい)かB(やや難しい)かを選択する。意欲ある方は、AとB両方を選択してもよい。学ぶ時間と、英会話力のレベルにより決定する。
2. CDを、細心の注意で複数回聞き、暗唱する。テキストを見ながらでもよい。(15分)
3. 各自、CDのネイティブ・スピーカーの発音をまね、左ページのAかBのダイアローグを声を出して読み、完全に暗記する。(15分)
4. 右ページに関しては、CDのネイティブ・スピーカーの発音に似せてリピートする。ここは、暗記というより、聞けば理解できるという程度でよい。(15分)
5. コラムを熟読し、医学知識を増やす。(5分)

● 英会話教師がいるクラス学習の場合…50分 or 90分

【クラスを担当する講師にお願い】

　１〜５までに関しては，基本的には前項（自習の場合）と同じでよい．ただし，時間配分は，少し短くなることに注意する．もし，90分授業であったなら，各課Ａ・Ｂの両方選択をお勧めする．前項と同じく，左ページは丸暗記が必須である．しかし右ページは，ヒヤリング中心でよい．講師の英文法に関する解説は，一切省略か，ほんの少しに限定する．(35分 or 60分)

６．クラスに数分間与え，左ページのダイアローグを暗記させる．(5分 or 10分)

７．クラスを２人ずつのペアに組ませ，左ページのダイアローグを対話形式で練習させる．役割を交替させ，各自に左ページすべての会話を暗記させる．(5分 or 10分)

８．代表のペアを複数組選び，クラスの前でダイアローグを暗唱させる．講師vs.全学生でダイアローグを再現してもよい．(5分 or 10分)

　本書の学習法のポイントは，左ページのダイアローグを，なるべくネイティブ・スピーカーの発音に似せて丸暗記することである．英会話授業であるので，この点を講師が強調してくれることを願いたい．

　英会話の第１歩は，ヒヤリングである．相手の喋ったことが理解できなければ，対話は成り立たない．アメリカ英語とイギリス英語の発音は違い，また，アメリカ英語にもイギリス英語にも，それぞれ地域語があり発音が相違する．どれが一番よいとは簡単に言えないが，発音の相違にもかかわらず，ネイティブ・スピーカー同士では，問題なく相互理解している．日本の文部科学省がアメリカ英語を選択しているので，本書はアメリカ標準英語の発音に従った．

　英会話は一夜では上達しない．学生は時間をかけ，コツコツと努力を積み上げることを期待されている．講師にとっては，そのために惜しみなく学生を励まし，勇気づけることが，大切な職務となっている．

2004年3月

植木 武　ドレール・トウン

To the English Instructors

Twenty years after we first published Practical English Conversation for Nurses, we are issuing this totally revised version to bring the content up to date and to make the language more accessible.

As before, the book is organized by chapters on outpatients and inpatients, portraying commonly seen situations in a variety of departments. A new addition is the section on care of the elderly at home and in care facilities. We have striven to make the conversations realistic—the type that nurses, in particular, but also doctors, technologists, dietitians, and other personnel encounter every day.

The book is characterized by the following:
1. The 25 chapters are divided into Lessons A and B, A usually being slightly easier.
2. Pronunciation of the medical terminology is that used in America and is indicated below the words in katakana.
3. Additional appropriate terms associated with each lesson's topic are given on the right-hand page.
4. Useful short sentences may also be provided on that page, mainly but not exclusively connected to that lesson's theme.
5. Under the heading "Column," interesting and useful facts about illnesses, as well as nurses and hospitals overseas, are given in Japanese only.

Hints for Using This Book
1. According to available class time (typically either 50 or 90 minutes) and the language ability of the students, Lessons A and B can be used alone or together.
2. The CD section for the left-page dialogue should be played two to three times as the students follow in their texts to familiarize them with a variety of voices. (Allow 10 minutes for 50-minute classes or 20 minutes for 90-minute classes.)
3. The instructor should then repeat the dialogue slowly with the students reciting together during the pauses. (Allow either 10 or 20 minutes.) This should be followed by 5 to 10 minutes of silent re-reading to memorize the lesson.
4. Playing the CD section for the right-hand page can be done more quickly since the students don't need to memorize the additional vocabulary, but they need to recognize

these terms when they hear them and be able to look them up. (8 or 15 minutes)

5. If the lesson has a Column on the right-hand page, give the students five minutes to read it. (5 minutes)

6. The instructor should then divide the students into pairs for role-playing using the dialogue. Halfway through, have them change roles. (10 or 15 minutes)

7. Finally, choose one or two pairs to do the dialogue one more time in front of the class. (5 or 10 minutes)

The first step to becoming at ease in foreign language conversation is hearing. Grasping what is being said must necessarily precede giving an answer. The English instructor may find the students very reluctant to speak up, even in answer to direct questions. Don't be daunted by this. Keep on talking! The important thing is to have their ears become accustomed to hearing your voice.

Differences in pronunciation between American and other English speakers and regional differences within America itself cannot all be addressed in one short text. We have chosen to go along with the standard American pronunciation in accordance with the choice of the Ministry of Education and Science.

Competence in English conversation is not acquired in a day or two. Repeated practice in listening and speaking gradually adds up to a useful skill. Your encouragement is a big part of that acquisition.

March 2004
Takeshi Ueki
Dorelle Toan

CONTENTS

Lesson 1-A あいさつ・自己紹介 1
　　　　　　Greetings, Introductions ……… 2
Vocabulary／いろいろなあいさつ Greetings

Lesson 1-B あいさつ・自己紹介 2
　　　　　　Greetings, Introductions ……… 4
Vocabulary／ちょっとした会話 Chats

Lesson 2-A 看護技術 1
　　　　　　Nursing Procedures ……… 6
Vocabulary／検査での表現 1／コラム

Lesson 2-B 看護技術 2
　　　　　　Nursing Procedures ……… 8
Vocabulary／検査での表現 2

Lesson 3-A 症状 1
　　　　　　Symptoms and Conditions ……… 10
Vocabulary／どんな状態？

Lesson 3-B 症状 2
　　　　　　Symptoms and Conditions ……… 12
Vocabulary／症状を訴える患者への対応

Lesson 4-A 受付にて
　　　　　　At Reception ……… 14
Vocabulary／専門科の名称を覚えよう！／初診患者に尋ねること

Lesson 4-B 会計
　　　　　　Billing ……… 16
Vocabulary／外来予約への対応／コラム

Lesson 5-A 風邪
　　　　　　Colds & Flu ……… 18
Vocabulary／風邪の症状を表現してみよう！

Lesson 5-B 胃の痛み
　　　　　　Stomachache ……… 20
Vocabulary／消化器系疾患の名前を覚えてみよう！／コラム

Lesson 6-A 内科―慢性腎不全
　　　　　　Internal Medicine－Chronic Renal Failure ……… 22
Vocabulary／覚えておきたい表現／コラム

Lesson 6-B 整形外科―関節症
　　　　　　Orthopedics－Joint Diseases ……… 24
Vocabulary／整形外科で使われる表現／コラム

Lesson 7-A 外科―胆石症
　　　　　　Surgery－Gallstones ……… 26
Vocabulary／痛みの表現 1

Lesson 7-B 外科―虫垂炎
　　　　　　Surgery－Appendicitis ……… 28
Vocabulary／痛みの表現 2／コラム

Lesson 8-A 小児科―喘息
　　　　　　Pediatrics－Asthma ……… 30
Vocabulary／子供に見られる症状や状態

Lesson 8-B 内科―摂食障害
　　　　　　Internal Medicine－Eating Disorders ……… 32
Vocabulary／気持ちを訴える患者…なんて答えよう？？？／コラム

Lesson 9-A 眼科―老人性白内障
　　　　　　Ophthalmology－Senile Cataracts ……… 34
Vocabulary／コラム

Lesson 9-B 耳鼻咽喉科―急性中耳炎
　　　　　　ENT－Acute Otitis Media ……… 36
Vocabulary／耳鼻咽喉科の症状を表現してみよう！

Lesson 10-A 皮膚科―アトピー性皮膚炎
　　　　　　Dermatology－Atopic Dermatitis ……… 38
Vocabulary／皮膚の状態を英語にしてみよう！

Lesson 10-B 泌尿器科―前立腺肥大症
　　　　　　Urology－Prostatic Hypertrophy ……… 40
Vocabulary／排泄の話

Lesson 11-A 産科―妊娠
　　　　　　Obstetrics－Pregnancy ……… 42
Vocabulary／産科で使われる表現／コラム

Lesson 11-B 放射線科―X線治療
　　　　　　Radiology Dept.－X-Ray Therapy ……… 44
Vocabulary／治療や病気、検査について患者はわかっているかしら？

Lesson 12-A 歯科―虫歯
　　　　　　Dentistry－Cavities ……… 46
Vocabulary／歯科で聞かれるフレーズを覚えよう！／コラム

Lesson 12-B 歯科―歯肉炎
　　　　　　Dentistry－Gingivitis ……… 48
Vocabulary／歯の状態を表現してみよう！

CONTENTS

Lesson 13-A 救命救急室―交通事故
　　　Emergency Room―Traffic Accident …… 50
　Vocabulary/救急でよく使われる表現１/コラム

Lesson 13-B 救急―心肺蘇生法
　　　Ambulance Call―Cardiopulmonary Resuscitation …… 52
　Vocabulary/救急でよく使われる表現２/コラム

Lesson 14-A 肺癌検査
　　　Lung Cancer Screening …… 54
　Vocabulary/X線検査での指示/コラム

Lesson 14-B 乳癌検査
　　　Breast Cancer Screening …… 56
　Vocabulary/婦人科で使われる表現

Lesson 15-A 心臓検査―ホルター心電図
　　　Cardiac Exam―Holter Monitor …… 58
　Vocabulary/検査についての説明をしてみよう！

Lesson 15-B 大腸検査
　　　Colonoscopy …… 60
　Vocabulary/検査中の患者への声かけ

Lesson 16-A 入院手続き
　　　Admission …… 62
　Vocabulary/病院内を案内してみよう！

Lesson 16-B 病室にて
　　　The Patient's Room …… 64
　Vocabulary/病棟を案内してみよう！

Lesson 17-A 脳卒中
　　　Stroke …… 66
　Vocabulary/脳卒中患者の様子

Lesson 17-B 心臓ペースメーカー
　　　Cardiac Pacemaker …… 68
　Vocabulary/循環器疾患をアセスメントしよう！/コラム

Lesson 18-A 手術の翌朝
　　　1st Morning Post-op …… 70
　Vocabulary/術前患者への説明

Lesson 18-B 術後3日
　　　3rd Day Post-op …… 72
　Vocabulary/術後患者への対応/コラム

Lesson 19-A 糖尿病
　　　Diabetes …… 74
　Vocabulary/糖尿病の症状とアドバイス

Lesson 19-B 退院指導
　　　Patient Teaching at Discharge …… 76
　Vocabulary/患者教育で使われるフレーズ/コラム

Lesson 20-A 足骨折
　　　Leg Fracture …… 78
　Vocabulary/リハビリが必要です！

Lesson 20-B 内分泌疾患―バセドウ病
　　　Endocrine Disorder―Graves' Disease …… 80
　Vocabulary/内分泌系をアセスメントしよう！/コラム

Lesson 21-A 陣痛と出産
　　　Labor and Delivery …… 82
　Vocabulary/不安いっぱい新米ママへの対応

Lesson 21-B 肝臓の病気
　　　Liver Disease …… 84
　Vocabulary/肝臓に問題のある患者をアセスメントしよう！

Lesson 22-A 肺炎
　　　Pneumonia …… 86
　Vocabulary/呼吸器疾患患者への対応

Lesson 22-B 骨粗鬆症
　　　Osteoporosis …… 88
　Vocabulary/日常生活についてアセスメントしてみよう！

Lesson 23-A 介護認定
　　　Care Designation …… 90
　Vocabulary/介護保険制度とは？/コラム

Lesson 23-B 在宅ケア―認知症
　　　Home Care―Dementia …… 92
　Vocabulary/薬の使い方を指示してみよう

Lesson 24-A 訪問介護―入浴サービス
　　　Home Care―Bath Service …… 94
　Vocabulary/日常介助のフレーズ

Lesson 24-B デイサービス
　　　Day Service …… 96
　Vocabulary/いろんな活動で話しかけてみよう

CONTENTS

Lesson 25-A 介護老人保健施設（老健）
Health Maintenance Nursing Home ···· 98
Vocabulary / よくある高齢者の訴え

Lesson 25-B 介護老人福祉施設（特養）
Long-Term Care Nursing Home ········ 100
Vocabulary / 褥瘡予防

資料　高齢者支援ネットワーク
Senior citizen's support Network ···· 102

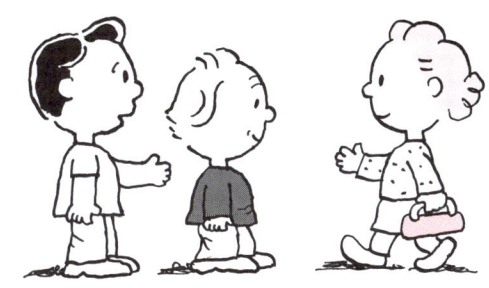

COLUMN

アメリカの病院におけるさまざまな看護師 ············· 7
アメリカの病院における患者の滞在期間 ············· 17
消化性潰瘍とピロリ菌 ··· 21
アメリカの病院で働く男性看護師に注目 ············· 23
関節リウマチと変形性関節症 ································· 25
いろいろな痛み ··· 29
摂食障害とは？ ··· 33
目の話 ··· 35
HIV/AIDSの深刻な話 ·· 43

耳よりな歯のはなし ··· 47
息子の臓器提供を励行したある夫妻の話 ············· 51
いろいろな傷 ··· 53
乳癌の早期発見と乳房温存手術 ····························· 55
ペースメーカーと携帯電話 ····································· 69
アメリカの病院で働く看護師が身につけるもの ···· 73
セラピューティック技術をマスターしよう！ ······ 77
急性肝炎について ··· 81
デイサービスとデイケアの違い ····························· 91

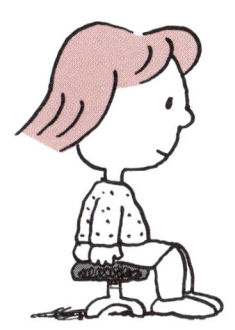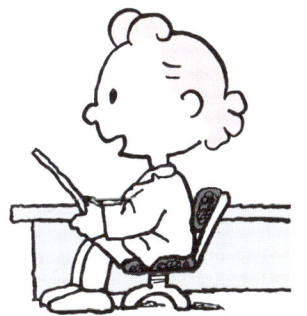

表紙／菊地慶矩　本文イラスト／望月恵子

ix

登場人物略語

AA = ambulance attendant

CE = city employee

CM = care manager

C = child

CA = cashier

D = doctor

DE = dentist

DH = dental hygienist

FM = family member

HH = home helper

H = helper

HB = husband

M = mother

MC = medical clerk

MT = medical technologist

N = nurse

P = patient

T = technologist

3rd Edition
Practical English Conversation for Nurses

看護英会話入門　第3版

Lesson 1-A

あいさつ・自己紹介1

Greetings, Introductions

N1：おはようございます．

N2：こんにちは．

N3：私は担当の看護師で，佐藤といいます．

N4：私は，ここの病棟師長をしている鈴木です．

▶ I'm Suzuki, the head nurse on this <u>floor</u>. という言い方もできる．「病棟」は一般にunitという．

 **Vocabulary をふやそう**　病院内スタッフ

| doctor, physician
ドクター　フィジィシャン | nurse
ナース | dentist
デンティストゥ | medical secretary
メディカル セクレタリー | unit secretary,
medical
office worker |

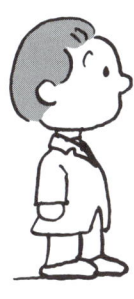 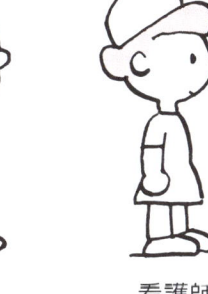 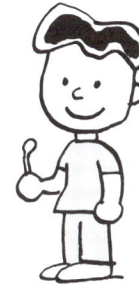 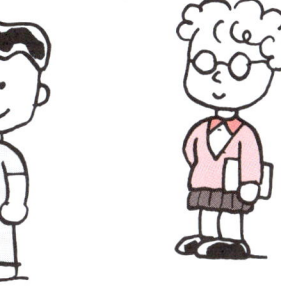 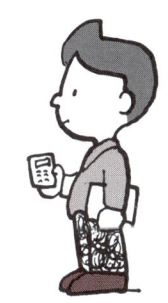

医師　　　　看護師　　　歯科医師　　　医療秘書　　　医療事務員

いろいろなあいさつ　Greetings

| Hi！ | Good morning. | How are you? | Bye,
see you tomorrow.
トゥモロー |

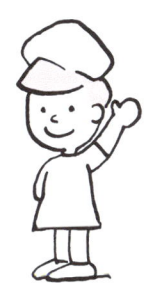 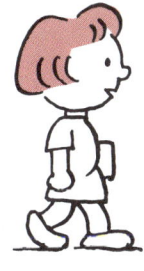 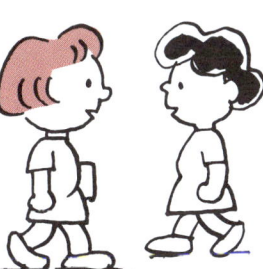  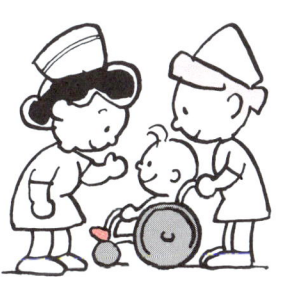

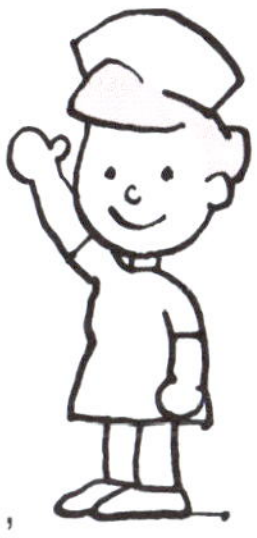

やぁ！　　　おはよう　　　　調子はどう？　　　　　じゃぁね，
また明日！

When are you next on nights?　　How do you do. I'm Takada.

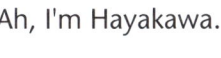Ah, I'm Hayakawa.

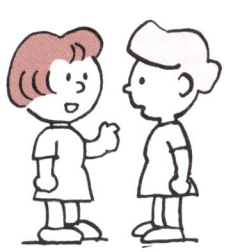 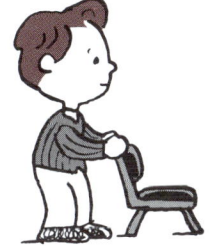 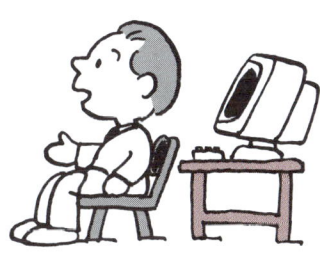

次の夜勤はいつ？　　　はじめまして，高田です．　　あっ，早川です．

Lesson 1-B

あいさつ・自己紹介2　Greetings, Introductions

Good evening.

N1：こんばんは．

How are you feeling?

N2：具合はいかがですか？

I'm a dental hygienist in the Dental Department.
ハイジェニストゥ

DH：私は歯科で働く歯科衛生士です．

I'm a medical technologist. I need to draw some blood.
ドゥロー
ブラッドゥ

MT：私は臨床検査技師で，採血をします．

 ## Vocabulary をふやそう　病院内スタッフ

medical engineer
メディカル　エンジニア

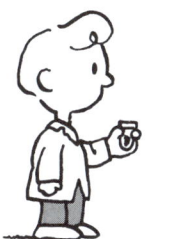

メディカルエンジニア

X-ray technician
エクスレイ　テクニシャン

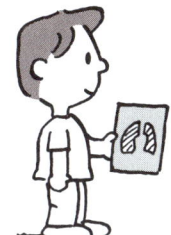

放射線技師

dietitian
ダイエティシャン

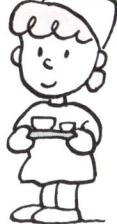

栄養士

occupational therapist
オキュペイショナル　セラピスト

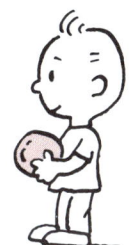

作業療法士

acupuncturist：鍼灸師
アキュパンクチュリストゥ

medical technologist：臨床検査技師
テクノロジィストゥ

physical therapist：理学療法士
セラピスト

pharmacist：薬剤師
ファーマスィストゥ

ちょっとした会話　Chats

The train stopped so I'm 15 minutes late.
ミニッツ

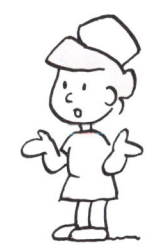

電車が止まって
15分の遅刻です．

Let's have lunch together.
トゥギャザー

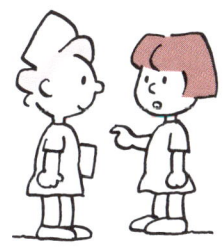

一緒にお昼ご飯を
食べましょう．

Dr. Mitsui has been looking for you.

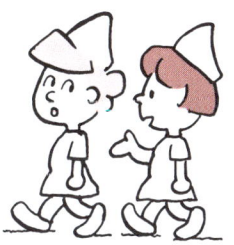

三井先生が
探していたよ．

When are you off?

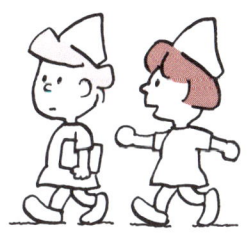

いつあがるの？

Do you want to go snowboarding over the New Year's holiday?

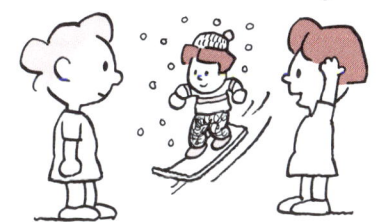

お正月休みにスノボーしに行く？

At six. How about dropping by somewhere?
　　　　　　　　　　　　　　　サムウェアー
6時よ．どこか寄って行かない？

Do you want to go to a beer garden after work?
仕事が終わったらビア・ガーデンに飲みに行かない？

Lesson 2-A

看護技術1

Nursing Procedures

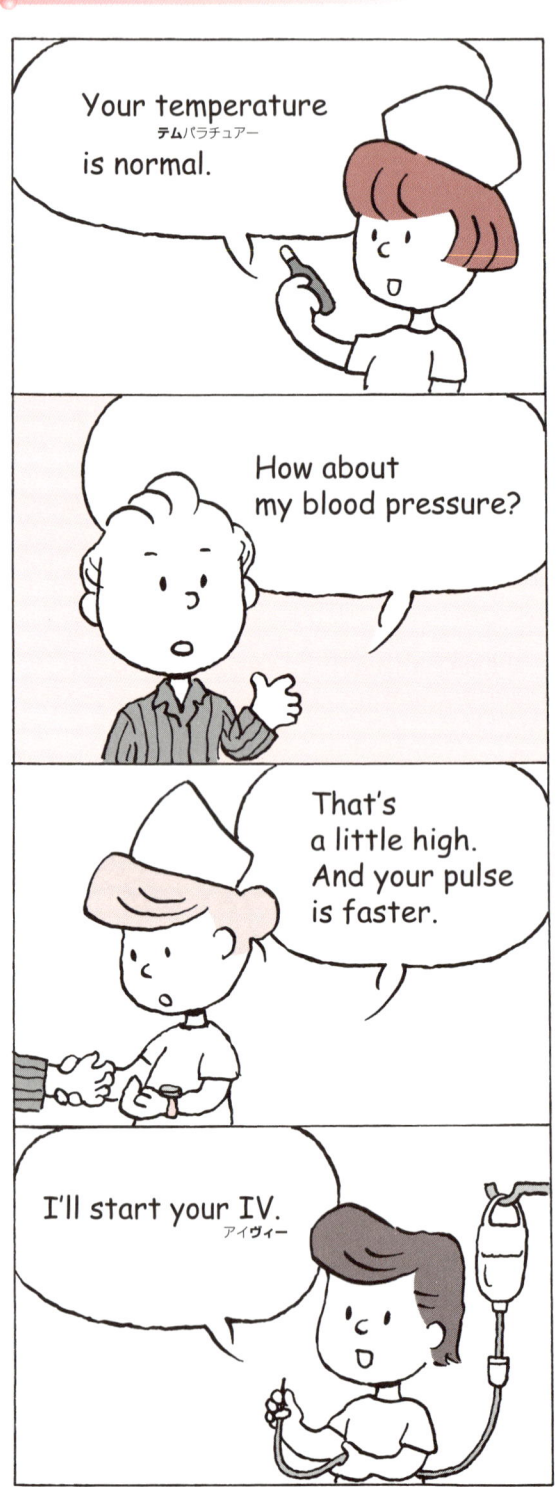

N1：平温ですよ．

P：血圧はどうですか？

☞ 血圧 blood pressure（ブラッド プレッシャー）はカルテなどではBPと略される．

N2：ちょっと高いですね．脈も速めです．

☞ 脈拍は pulse（パルス）．「脈をみる」は check the pulse，「脈をとる」は take one's pulse という．

N3：点滴をしましょう．

☞ IV は intravenous（イントゥラヴィーナス）のことで，静脈（内）注射，点滴静注を示す．点滴はIV drip ともいう．

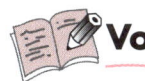 ## Vocabulary をふやそう　病院内機器

thermometer	blood pressure gauge,	drip infusion kit	endoscope	electrocardiogram
サーモメター	sphygmomanometer	インフュージョン	エンドスコウプ	エレクトゥロカーディオグラム
	ゲイジュ／スフィグモマナメター			（ECGまたはEKG）

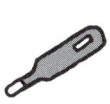 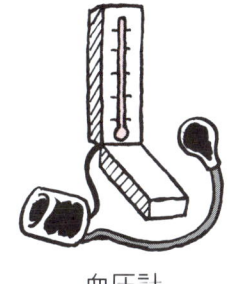 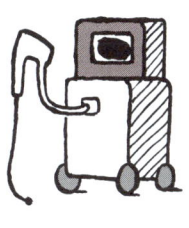 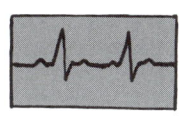

体温計　　　血圧計　　　点滴装置　　　内視鏡　　　心電図

検査での表現 1

| Would you step on the scale? | I'll check your blood pressure. | Please collect a urine sample in this cup.　ユーリン　サンプル |

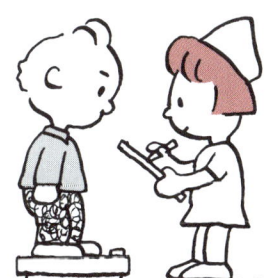 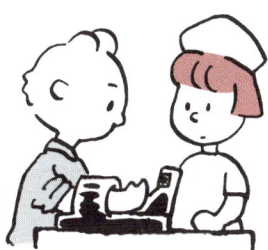 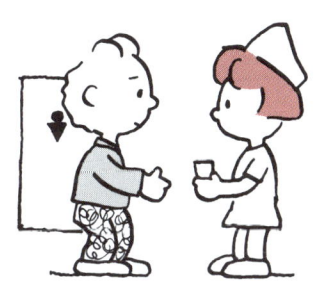

体重計にのって下さい．　　血圧を測りますよ．　　このカップに尿のサンプルを採ってください．

COLUMN アメリカの病院におけるさまざまな看護師　American Nursing Hierarchy

Director of Nursing：看護部長，総師長
Nursing Supervisor：看護副部長，複数の病棟の責任者
Head Nurse：看護師長，病棟責任者
R.N.（Registered Nurse）：登録看護師
L.P.N.／L.V.N.：Licensed Practical NurseまたはLicensed Vocational Nurseの略．1年制プログラム卒の看護師のこと．

Lesson 2-B

看護技術2

Nursing Procedures

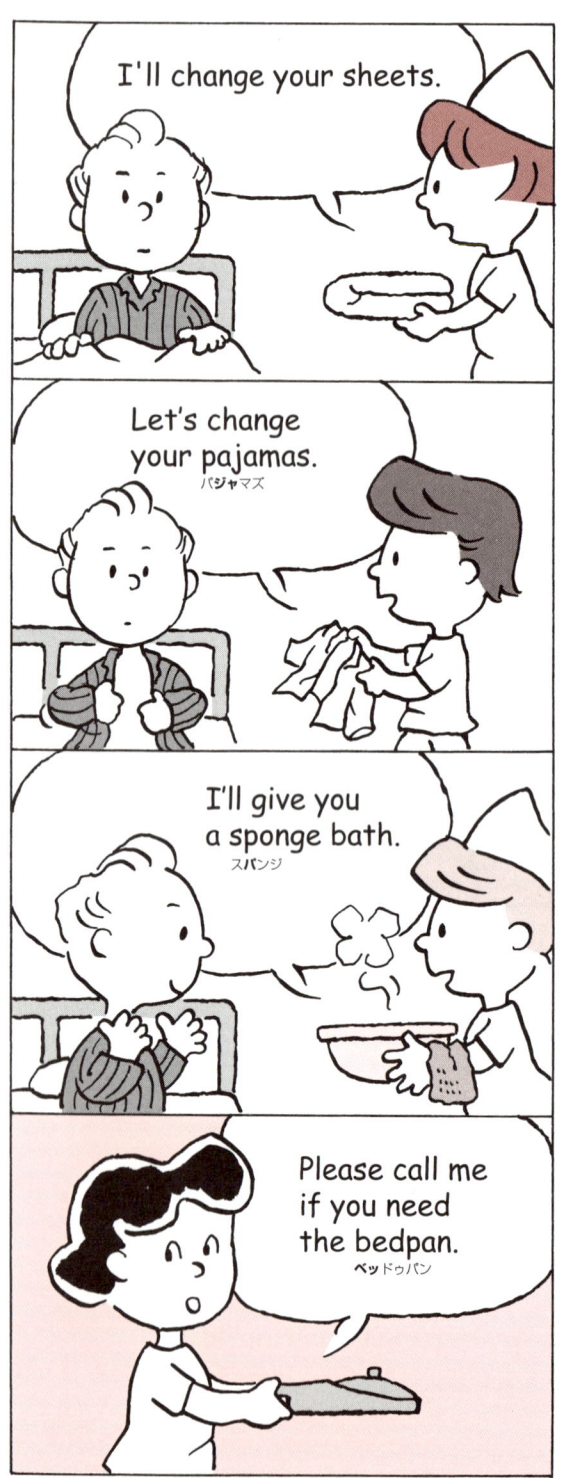

N1：シーツの交換をしましょう．

N2：パジャマを換えましょう．

N3：体を拭きましょう．

☞ a sponge bath は清拭ともいう．

N4：便器が必要なときは
　　 呼んでくださいね．

📖 Vocabulary をふやそう

portable toilet

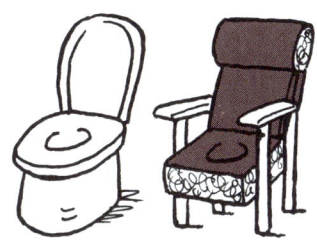

ポータブル便器

urinal
ユリナル

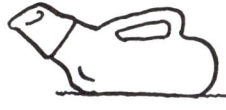

尿瓶

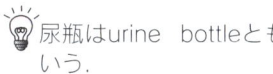
💡 尿瓶はurine bottleともいう．

gown

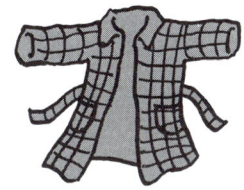

ガウン

towel：タオル

soap：石鹸
ソウプ

shampoo：シャンプー
💡 シャンプーとセットに考えられているリンスrinseは「すすぐ，洗い落とす」という意味もある．

bedpan：便器
ベッドゥパン

🔲 検査での表現 2 🔲

I'll get a blood sample.
Please sit here
and roll up your sleeve.

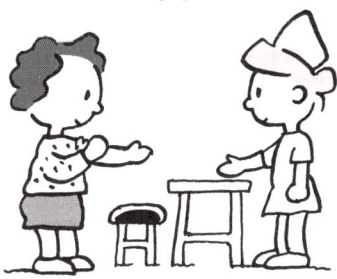

採血をします．
ここに座って，
袖を上げてください．

Make a tight fist...
All right, now you can relax.

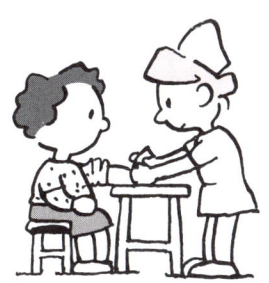

きつくこぶしを握ってください．
もうリラックスしていいですよ．

Press this to
your arm until
the bleeding stops.

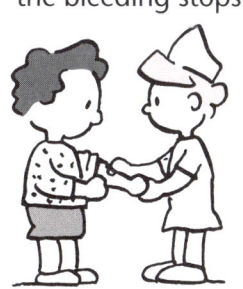

出血が止まるまで，
これで押さえて
おいてください．

When you have a bowel movement, please collect a sample in this container.
　　　　　　　　　　バウル　ムーブメントゥ　　　　　　　　　　　　　　カンテイナー
A small amount is okay.
　　　　アマウントゥ

排便の後にサンプルを取り，この中に入れてください．少量で結構です．

Lesson 3-A

症状1

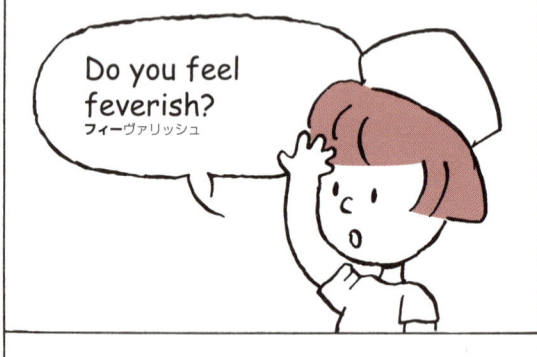

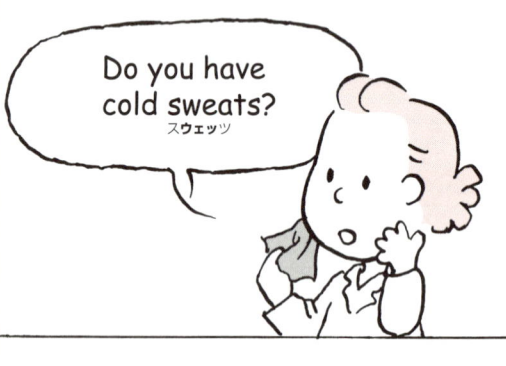

Symptoms and Conditions

I feel weak.

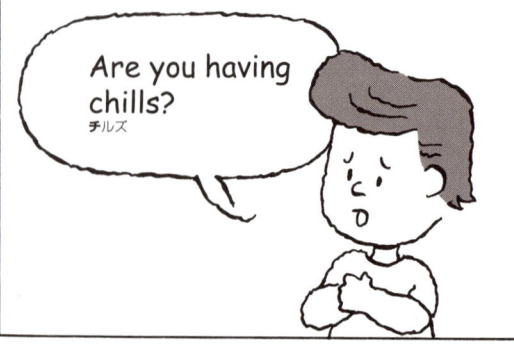

P：力が入りません．

Do you feel feverish?
フィーヴァリッシュ

N1：熱があるようですか？

☞ feverish は「熱っぽい，ほてる」という意味．

Do you have cold sweats?
スウェッツ

D：冷や汗が出ますか？

Are you having chills?
チルズ

N2：悪寒がしていますか？

 ## vocabulary をふやそう

weakness
ウィークネス
だるい，脱力感

chest pain
チェスト　ペイン
胸痛，
胸が苦しい状態

dehydration
ディハイドレイション
脱水状態

fever, elevated temperature
フィーヴァー　エレヴェイティドゥ
テムパラチュアー
発熱

dizziness, vertigo
ディズィネス　ヴァーティゴウ
めまい

sweat, perspiration
スウェットゥ　パースピレイション
発汗

paleness, pallor
ペイルネス　パーラー
顔面蒼白

tinnitus, ringing in the ears
ティニタス
耳鳴

 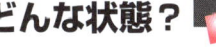 ## どんな状態？

I'm thirsty.
サースティー

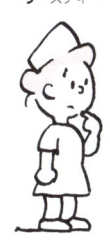

のどが
渇いています．

My face looks pale.
ペイル

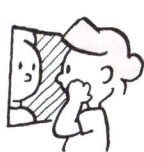

顔色が悪いです．

I'm hungry.
ハングリー

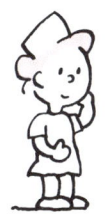

おなかが
すいています．

I'm sleepy.

眠いです．

I'm tired.
タイアードゥ

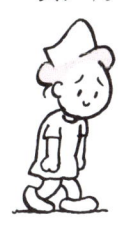

疲れています．

I feel nauseated.
ノーズィエイティドゥ

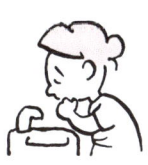

吐き気がします．

I have a fever.
フィーヴァー

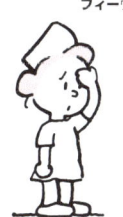

熱があります．

I have stiff shoulders.
スティフ

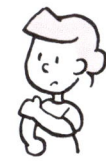

肩がこっています．

I feel short of breath.
ブレス
息切れしています．

I feel faint.
フェイント
めまいがします．

I feel a little cold.
少し寒いです．

I need to go to bathroom.
トイレに
行きたいです．

My legs feel weak / heavy.
ヘヴィー
足がだるいです．

I want to sit down.
座りたいです．

Ouch!
アウチ
痛い！

I have a headache.
ヘデエイク
頭が痛いです．

Lesson 3-B

症状2　Symptoms and Conditions

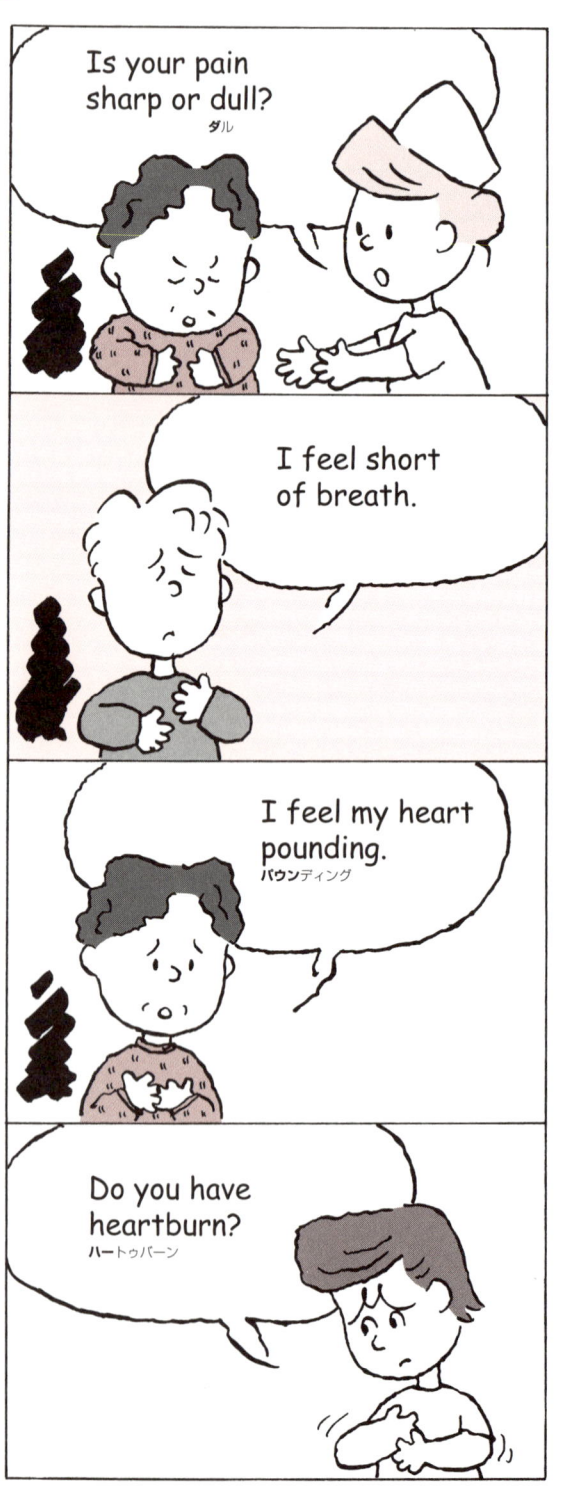

N1：鋭い痛みですか？それとも鈍痛ですか？

P1：息切れがします．

☞「息が苦しい」なら I have trouble breathing.

P2：心臓がどきどきします．

☞ I have palpitations.（パルピテイションズ）ともいう．palpitation は「動悸，胸騒ぎ」の意．

N2：胸やけがしますか？

Vocabulary をふやそう

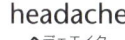 headache
ヘデェエイク

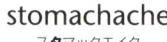 stomachache
スタマックエイク

rash
ラッシュ

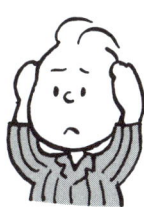
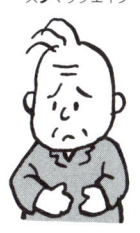
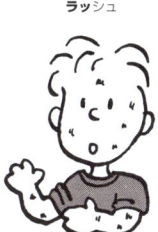

頭痛　　　　　胃痛　　　　　発疹

throbbing pain：疼痛，ずきずきする痛み
スラビィング

vomiting, emesis：嘔吐
ヴァーミティング　エメスィス

passing gas：おならをすること
ギャス

hives：じんま疹
ハイヴス

fainting, syncope：失神
フェインティング　スィンクピ

症状を訴える患者への対応

P：I'm always constipated. ［←レッスン３A（11頁）の表現などを使ってみましょう！］
　　カンスティペイティドゥ
　　いつも便秘がちです．

N：When was your last bowel movement?
　　　　　　　　　　　バウル
　　最後にお通じがあったのはいつですか？

P：About five days ago.
　　5日ほど前です．

N：Let's talk with the doctor about a laxative (a change of diet).
　　　　　　　　　　　　　　　　　ラクサティヴ
　　医師に下剤のことを相談してみましょう（食事療法について相談してみましょう）．

P：Can't I have an enema?
　　　　　　　　　エネマ
　　浣腸してくれませんか？

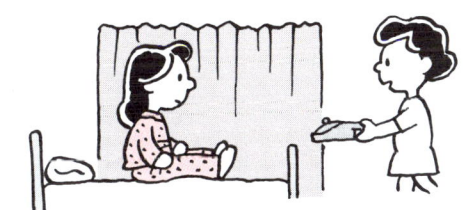

Lesson 4-A

受付にて / At Reception

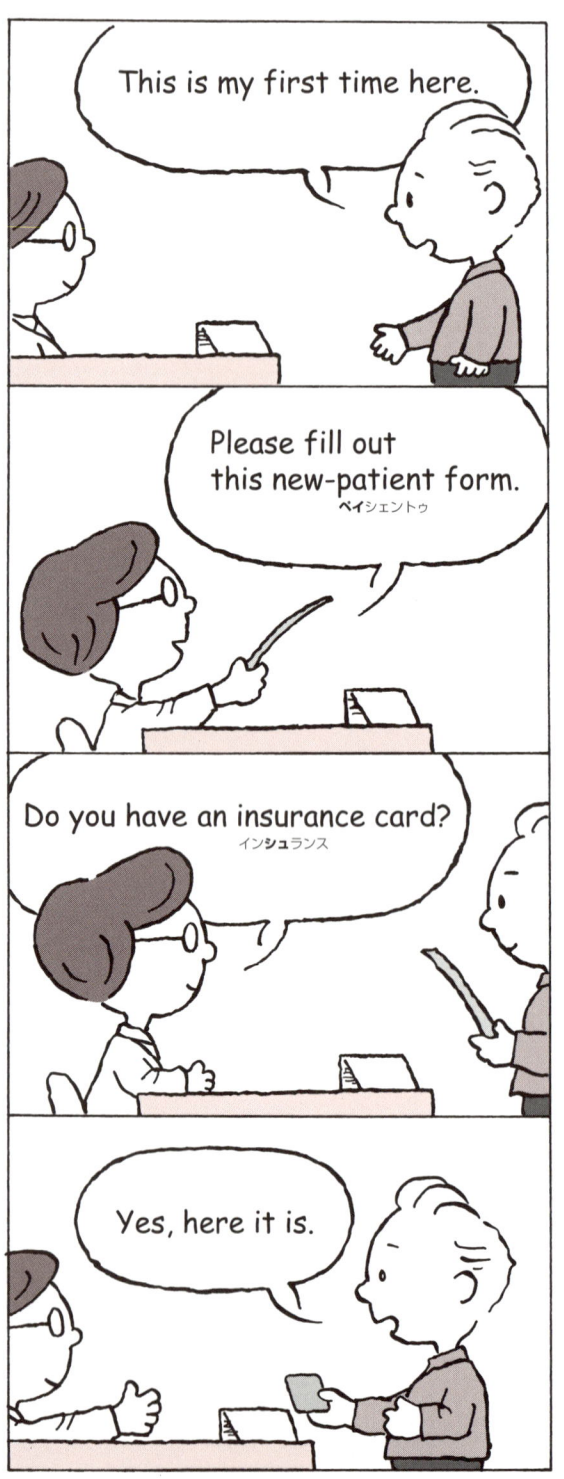

P：初めて来ました．

MC：どうぞ，初診用書類に書き込んでください．

MC：保険証をお持ちですか？

P：はい，ここにあります．

Vocabulary をふやそう

medical history form：問診票
　ヒストゥリー フォーム
national health insurance：国民健康保険
number ticket：番号札

patient card, consultation card
カンサルテイション

chart
チャートゥ

insurance card

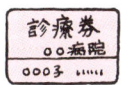
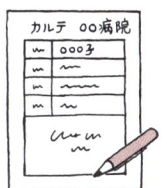
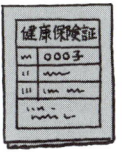

診察カード　　　カルテ　　　保険証

専門科の名称を覚えよう！

内科：internal medicine
　　　インターナル メディスン
外科：surgery
　　　サージェリー
整形外科：orthopedics
　　　　　オーソピーディックス
皮膚科：dermatology
　　　　ダーマタロジー
眼科：ophthalmology
　　　アフサルマロジー
耳鼻科：ENT（ear, nose and throat）

産婦人科：obstetrics and gynecology（OB-Gyn）
　　　　　アブステトリックス　　ガイネカロジー
小児科：pediatrics
　　　　ピディアトゥリックス
神経科：neurology
　　　　ニューラロジー
精神科：psychiatry
　　　　サイカエトゥリー
泌尿器科：urology
　　　　　ユーラロジー

初診患者に尋ねること

Can I ask your _____?　下線部に次の言葉を入れて言ってみよう.
・氏名，住所，電話番号：name, address, telephone number
・体重，身長：weight, height　・生年月日：birth date

Do you have _____?　下線部に次の言葉を入れて言ってみよう.
・しっしんやかぶれ：a rash　・喘息：asthma　・じんま疹：hives
　　　　　　　　　　　　　　　　アズマ　　　　　　　　　ハイヴズ

その他のフレーズ
・注射や薬で調子が悪くなったことがありますか？：
　　Have you had a bad reaction to an injection or other medication?
・重い病気をしたことがありますか？：Have you had any major medical problems?
・現在，薬を飲んでいますか？：Are you currently taking any medication?
・今，妊娠中ですか？： Are you now pregnant?
・子供のころ（病名）にかかったことがありますか？
　　Have you had _____ when you were a child?
　　　・はしか：measles　・風疹：German measles　・水疱瘡：chicken pox
　　　　　　　　ミーズルズ　　　　　　ジャーマン　　　　　　　　　　　　パックス
　　　・おたふく風邪：mumps　・自家中毒：autotoxemia
　　　　　　　　　　　マムプス　　　　　　　オートタクスィミア

15

Lesson 4-B

会計 / Billing

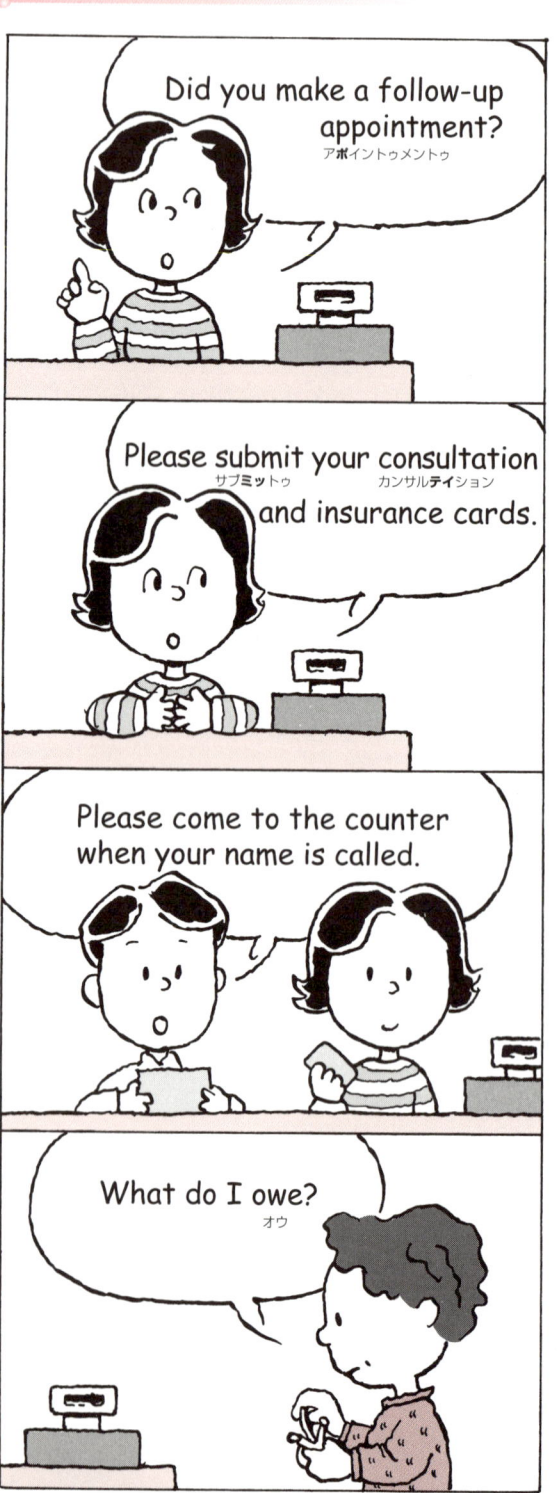

CA：次回の予約をとりましたか？

CA：診察券と保険証をご提出ください．

CA：お名前を呼ばれたらカウンターまでお越しください．

P：おいくらですか？

☞ How much is it? でも可．

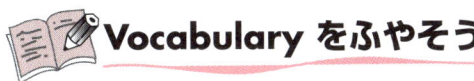 Vocabulary をふやそう

cashier：会計窓口

bill, list of charges：請求書
チャージズ

receipt：領収書
リスィートゥ

appointment slip：予約票
スリップ

prescription：処方箋
プリスクリプション

parking lot ticket：駐車チケット
パーキング ラットゥ ティケットゥ

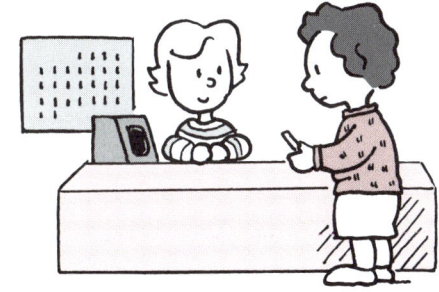

外来予約への対応

P：Dr. Takahashi in Surgery said I should come back in one month.
　　　　　　サージェリー
外科の高橋先生が，1か月後に来るようにと言われました．

C：Dr. Takahashi is here on Mondays and Thursdays.
高橋先生は月曜と木曜にいらっしゃいますよ．

P：I can come on Thursday, June 20th.
6月20日の木曜なら大丈夫です．

C：Do you want a morning or an afternoon appointment?
午前の予約にしますか，それとも午後にしますか？

COLUMN アメリカの病院における患者の滞在期間　Length of Stay in the Hospital

アメリカでは，入院期間が非常に短いです．盲腸炎（appendicitis），ヘルニア（hernia），白内障（cataract）などの手術は外来で行われるので，朝，病院に入り，夕食のころには自宅に帰れます．扁桃摘出術（tonsillectomy）も，痛みが激しい，嚥下（swallow）ができないなどの問題がなければ，日帰りです．出産（delivery）は通常なら二晩泊まりまでです．

Lesson 5-A

風邪   Colds & Flu

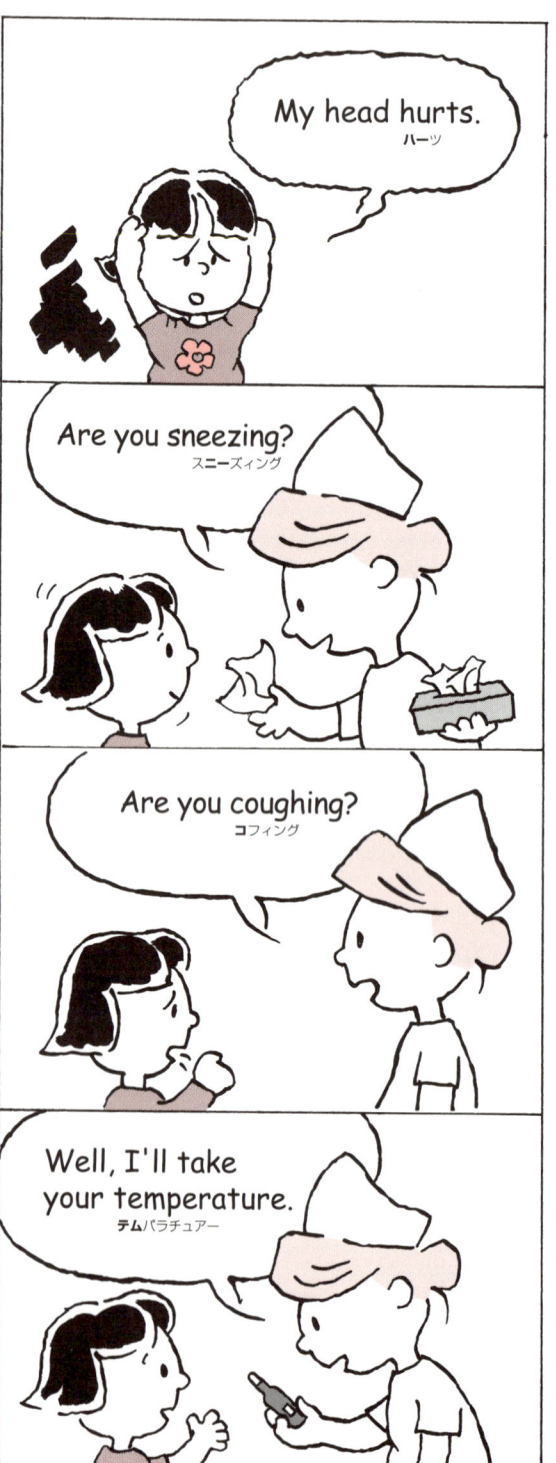

C：頭が痛いです．

☞ I have a headache. は「(ここのところ)頭が痛い」という意味で，「ある程度の時間，頭痛を抱えている」というニュアンスである．一方，My head hurts. は「(今)頭が痛い」というニュアンスである．

N1：くしゃみが出ますか？

N2：咳が出ていますか？

N3：では熱を測りましょう．

☞ I'll see if you have a fever. とも言える．

 **Vocabulary** をふやそう

cold：風邪，感冒
コウルドゥ

influenza：インフルエンザ　💡 略して，flu：フルーとも言う．

sore throat：咽頭痛
ソーアー スロウトゥ

sinusitis：副鼻腔炎（蓄膿症）
サイナスアイティス

(chronic) bronchitis：(慢性)気管支炎
クロニック　ブロンカイティス

pneumonia：肺炎
メーモウニア

viral infection：ウイルス感染
ヴァイラル インフェクション

風邪の症状を表現してみよう！

I have a runny nose.　　I have a cough.　　I'm feeling chilly.　　I'm feeling sluggish.
　ラニー　　　　　　　　　コフ　　　　　　　　チリー　　　　　　　スラギッシュ

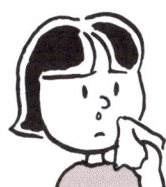 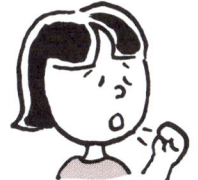 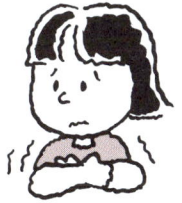 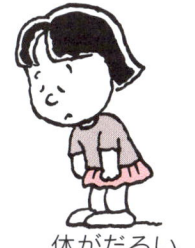

鼻水が出る．　　　　　咳が出る．　　　　　悪寒がする．　　　　　体がだるい．

　　💡 どれも I'm suffering from で置き換えられる．

I have a stuffy nose.
　　スタフィー
　鼻が詰まる．

I have a sore throat.
　　ソーアー スロウトゥ
　喉が痛い．

I have (a slight / a high) fever.
　　　　スライトゥ
　（微熱／高熱）が出ている．

I'm sneezing.
　スニーズィング
　くしゃみが出る．

19

Lesson 5-B

胃の痛み

Stomachache

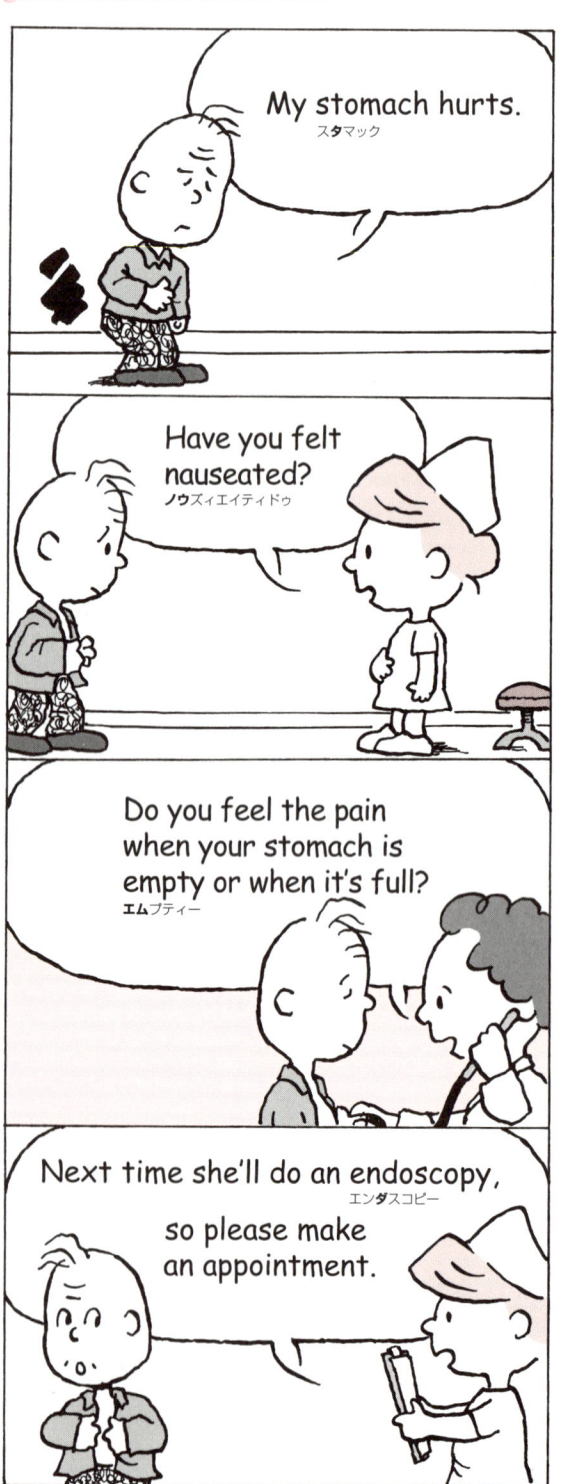

P：胃が痛むんです．

N：吐き気はありますか？

D：痛みは空腹時ですか？それとも食後ですか？

N：次回は内視鏡検査がありますので，予約してください．

Vocabulary をふやそう

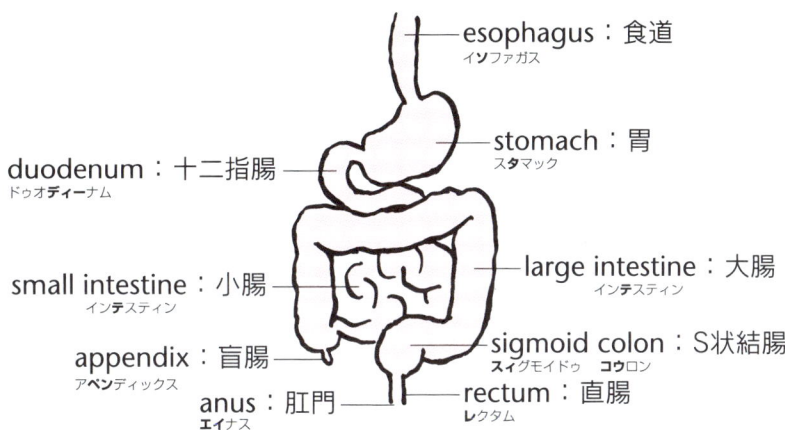

消化器系疾患の名前を覚えてみよう！

stomach ulcer：胃潰瘍
アルサー

gastritis：胃炎
ギャストゥライティス

duodenal ulcer：十二指腸潰瘍
ドゥオディーノル アルサー

esophageal reflux：食道逆流
イサファジール リフラックス

colon cancer：大腸癌
コウロン キャンサー

rectal cancer：直腸癌
レクタル

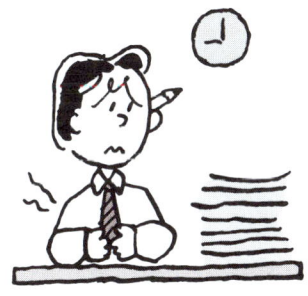

COLUMN 消化性潰瘍とピロリ菌 Peptic Ulcers and *H. Pylori*

消化性潰瘍と呼ばれる胃・十二指腸潰瘍は，ヘリコバクター・ピロリ菌（*Helicobacter pylori*）との関係が明らかになっています．胃液中胃酸により胃内では細菌が生息できないと考えられていましたが，電子顕微鏡（**electron microscope**）によってピロリ菌がいることがわかりました．抗生物質（**antibiotic**）で除菌すると胃・十二指腸潰瘍が治ったり，再発しなくなることが臨床的に証明されています．しかし，アスピリンなど薬剤が原因で起こるもの（**drug-induced**）はピロリ菌がいなくても潰瘍が生じます．

Lesson 6-A

内科-慢性腎不全

Internal Medicine - Chronic Renal Failure

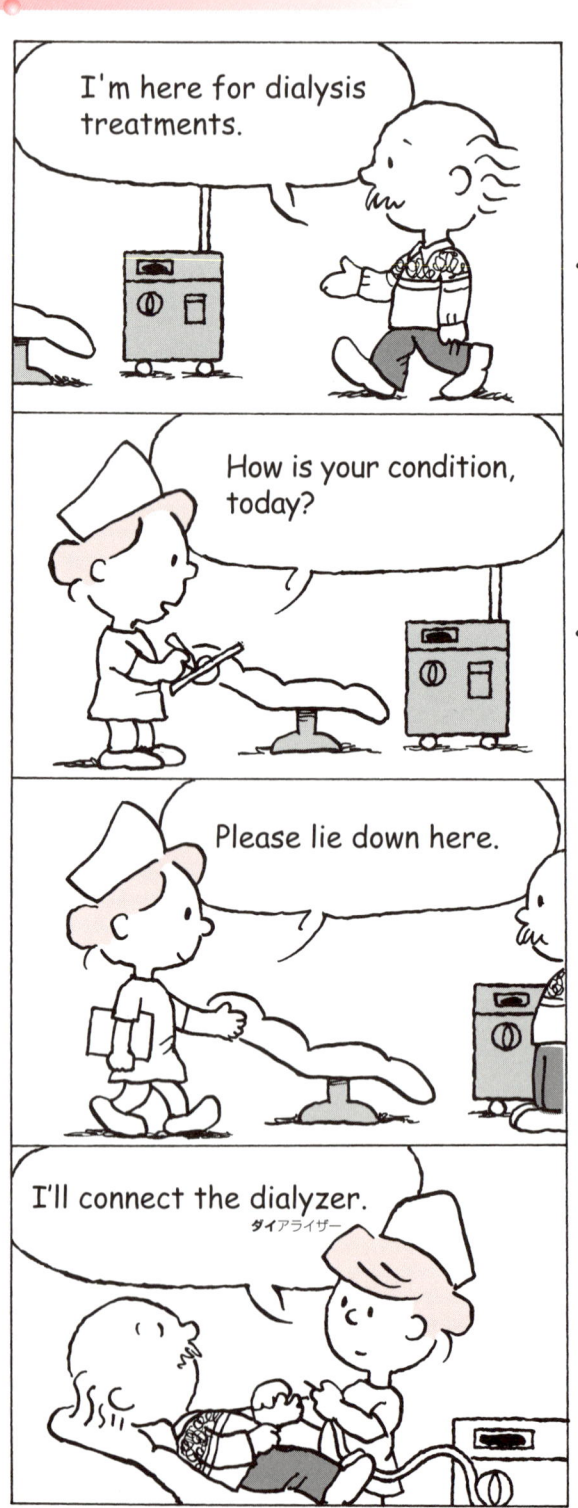

P：人工透析に来ました．

☞ hemodialysis（血液透析）のこと．略語はHD．

N：今日の体調はいかがですか？

☞ この場合，How are you feeling today？でも良い．

N：ここに横になってください．

N：透析器をつなぎます．

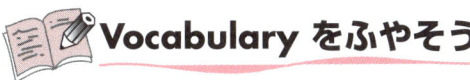 Vocabulary をふやそう

kidney：腎臓
キドゥニー

cystitis：膀胱炎
スィスタイティス

acute nephritis：急性腎炎
アキュートゥ ネフライティス

renal/kidney transplant：腎移植
リーナル　　　　　トゥランスプラントゥ

urinalysis：尿検査
ユリナリスィス

edema：浮腫
エディーマ

forced fluids：強制輸液
フォーストゥ フルーイッズ

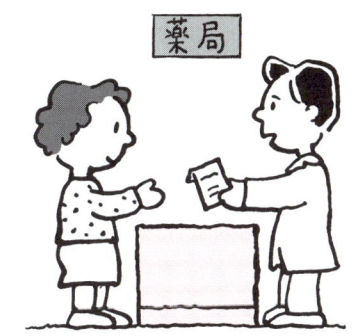

pharmacyは処方薬のみを扱う薬局のこと．drugstoreは常備薬や日常雑貨を扱っているが，よく一隅に薬剤師のいるpharmacyを有する．

覚えておきたい表現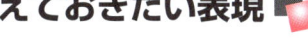

週2回：twice a week

1日3回：three times a day

1回5時間：five hours each time

毎食後：after each meal

寝る前に：before going to sleep

空腹時に：on an empty stomach
　　　　　　　　　　　スタマック

医師の指示どおりに：according to doctor's instructions

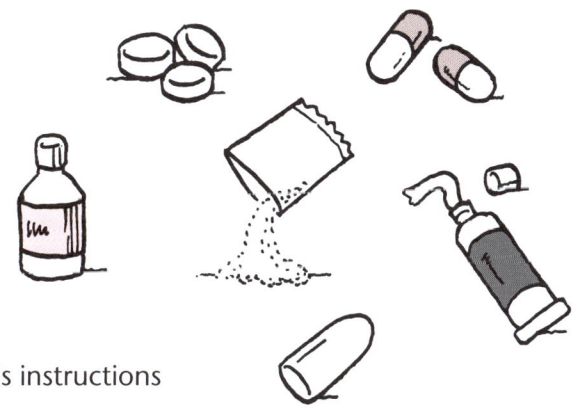

COLUMN　アメリカの病院で働く男性看護師に注目　American Male Nurses

アメリカでは，病院によって違いますが，男性看護師はだいたい1割強を占めています．男性看護師は救急室（ER, emergency room），集中治療室（ICU, intensive care unit），開胸病棟（open-heart unit），麻酔室（anesthesia room）などで働き，一般病棟にはあまり行かない傾向にあります．

Lesson 6-B

整形外科 – 関節症
Orthopedics – Joint Diseases

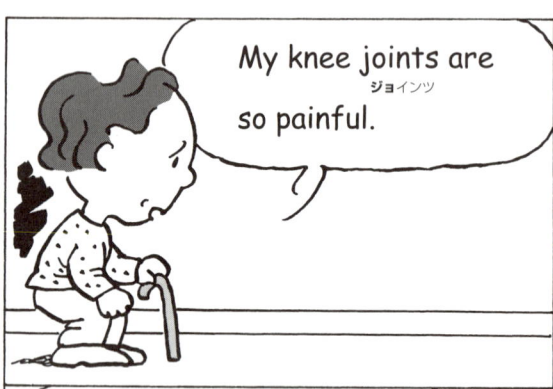

P：膝の関節がとても痛いです．

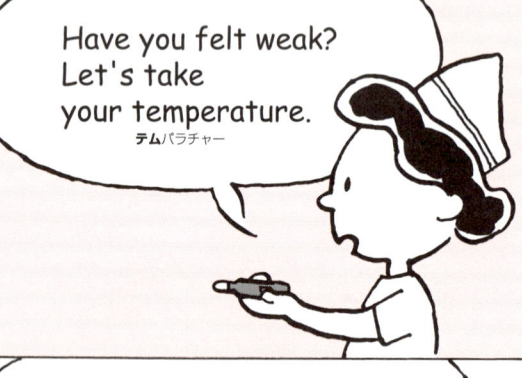

N：脱力感がありますか？
　　熱を測りましょう．

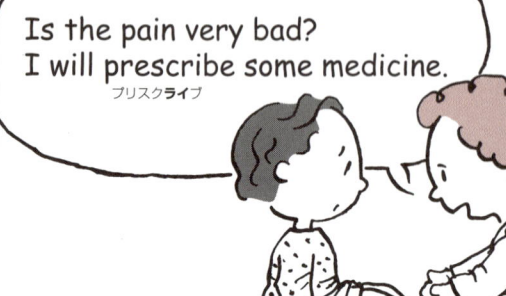

D：かなり痛いですか？ 薬を
　　出しておきましょう．

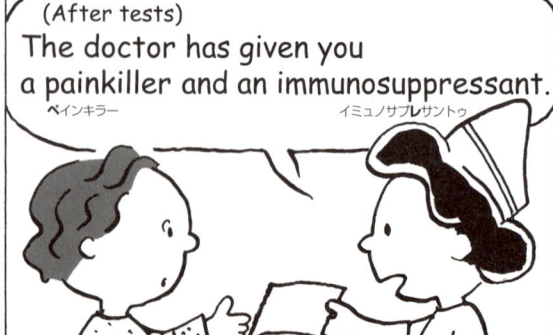

(検査後)

N：先生から痛み止めと免疫抑制剤が
　　処方されましたよ．

☞ pain（痛み）＋killer（殺し屋）で「痛み止め」，
immune（免疫）＋suppressant（抑制）で「免疫抑制剤」，
医療英語には複合語が多い．

Vocabulary をふやそう

arthritis：関節炎
アースライティス

osteoarthritis：変形性関節症
アスティオアースライティス

swelling, enlargement：腫脹
スウェリング　エンラージメントゥ

morning stiffness：朝のこわばり
スティフネス

inflammation：炎症
インフラメイション

deformity：変形
ディフォーミティー

整形外科で使われる表現

I have a fracture.
フラクチュアー
骨折しています．

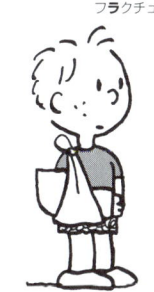

I have low back pain.
腰痛があります．

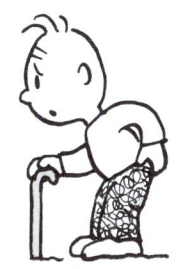

I have difficulty walking.
歩行が困難です．

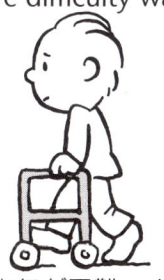

I have had dislocations of the joints.
ディスロケイションズ　ジョインツ
関節脱臼を起こしたことがあります．

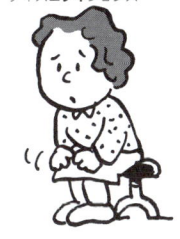

COLUMN 関節リウマチと変形性関節症　Rheumatoid Arthritis vs. Osteoarthritis
ルーマトイドゥ　アースライティス

関節リウマチ（RA）は，膠原病（collagen disease）の一つに分類されます．免疫性の病気で，滑膜炎（synovitis）が起こり，そこから関節軟骨や骨が溶けていく病気です．変形性関節炎（OA）は，関節が繰り返し使用され軟骨がすり減り，そのため軟骨が自己増殖しようとするのです．つまり，磨耗と自己増殖が同時に行われている状態です．40〜50代から，膝（knee），指（finger），股関節（hip joint），足首（ankle），背骨（spine），肘（elbow）などに発症し，女性は男性より10倍多いです．RAとOAの相違は，RAは20〜50歳の間に突然発病し，両側の関節が同時に腫れたりほてったり（炎症）し，全身のだるさや疲労感，体重減少，発熱を伴うのに対し，OAは長年にわたり病状が進行し，たいてい40歳以降に発症し，体の片側の関節に症状が現れ，しかし，発熱や体全体のだるさはありません．

Lesson 7-A

外科-胆石症

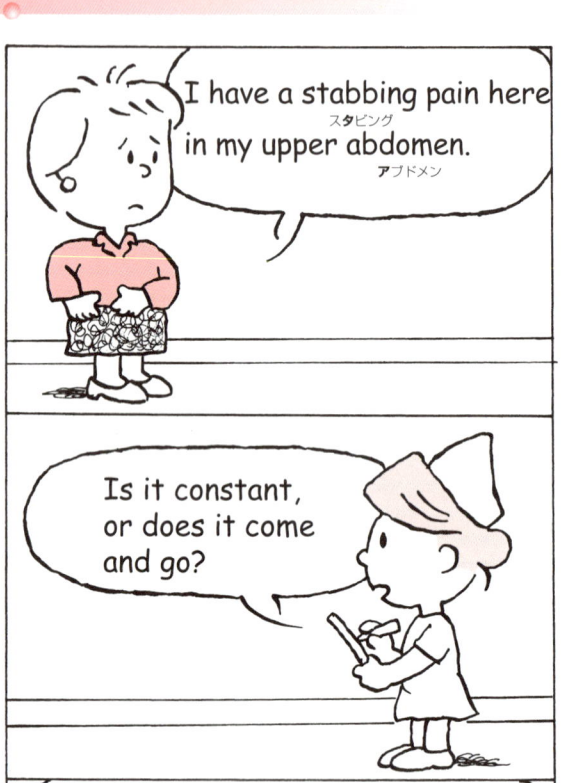

Surgery-Gallstones

I have a stabbing pain here in my upper abdomen.
スタビング　アブドメン

P：おなかの上のほうに差し込むような痛みがあります．

☞ abdomen は腹部全体を指す単語．

Is it constant, or does it come and go?

N：ずっと痛みますか，それともときどき痛みますか？

Well, it comes on after heavy, oily meals. I hope it isn't cancer.
キャンサー

P：えーっと，脂っこい食事をとると痛みます．癌じゃないでしょうね．

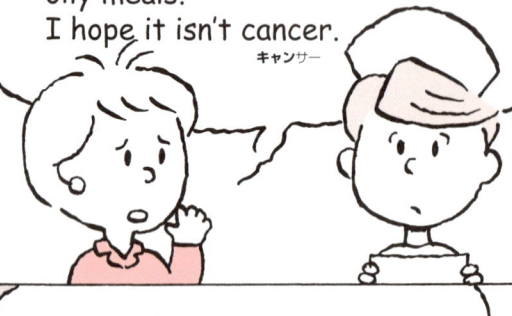

Your problem is probably gallstones. Let's get some x-rays and an ultrasound test.
ゴールストゥンズ　　　　アルトゥラサウンドゥ

D：胆石かもしれません．X線と超音波検査をしましょう．

☞ 超音波検査(ultrasound test)は，エコー検査(echo test)ともいう．

📝 Vocabulary をふやそう

red blood cell, erythrocyte：赤血球
　　　　　セル　　エリスロサイトゥ

white blood cell, leukocyte：白血球
　　　　　　　　　　ルコサイトゥ

bile：胆汁
バイル

stone, calculus：結石
　　　　キャルキュラス

cholangiogram：胆管造影
コランジオグラム

gallbladder：胆嚢
ゴールブラダー

differential diagnosis：鑑別診断
　　　　　　ダイアグノウスィス

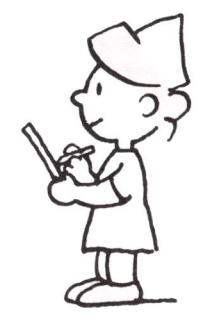

痛みの表現 1

sharp pain

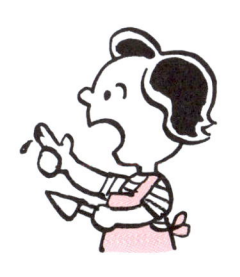

鋭い痛み

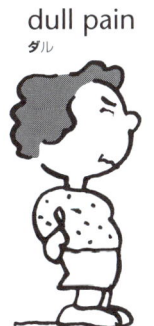

dull pain
ダル

鈍い痛み

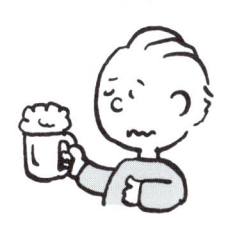

burning pain

焼けるような痛み

pressing pain

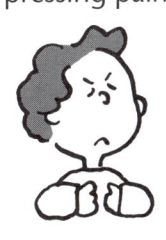

締めつけられるような痛み

stinging pain：ヒリヒリする痛み
スティンイング

colicky pain：疝痛（腹部の痙攣痛）
カリキー

Lesson 7-B

外科-虫垂炎

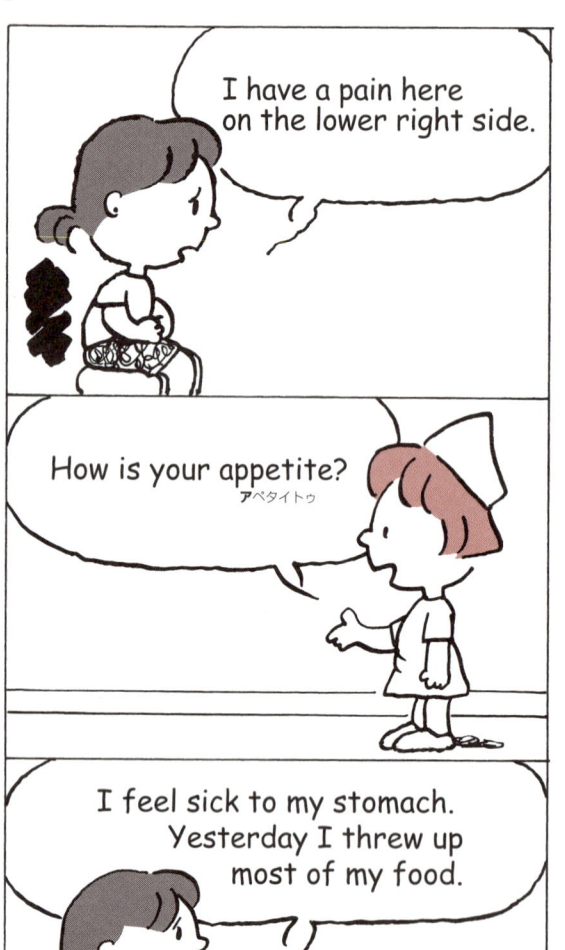

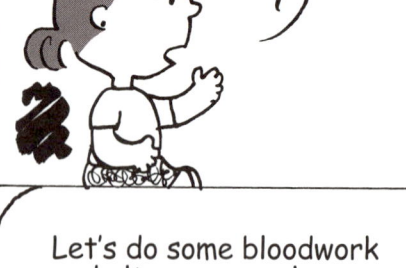

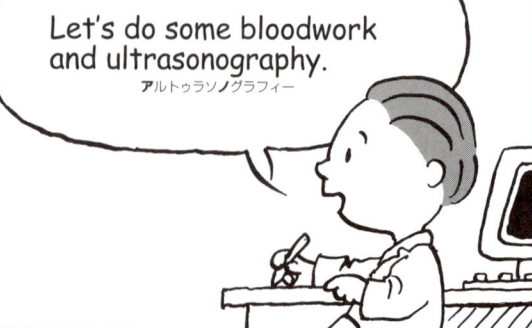

Surgery-Appendicitis

I have a pain here on the lower right side.

P：右の下のほうが痛みます．

How is your appetite?
アペタイトゥ

N：食欲はどうですか？

I feel sick to my stomach. Yesterday I threw up most of my food.

P：胃がむかむかします．昨日は食べたものをほとんど吐いてしまいました．

☞「胃がむかむかする（吐き気がする）」は I feel nauseated. という言い方もある.
ノーズィエイティドゥ

Let's do some bloodwork and ultrasonography.
アルトゥラソノグラフィー

D：血液検査と超音波検査をしましょう．

☞「超音波検査（エコー検査）」は，空洞の腹部に音波を与え，こだましたものを画面に映すことから echo と呼ばれる．

Vocabulary をふやそう

nausea：吐き気
ノーズィア

vomiting：嘔吐
ヴァーミティング

referred pain：関連痛
リファードゥ

rupture：破裂
ラプチュアー

lumbar anesthesia：腰椎麻酔
ランバー　　アネススィージア

loss of sensation：感覚喪失
センセイション

liquid diet：流動食
リクィドゥ

bowel sounds：腸音
バウル

痛みの表現 2

piercing pain
ピアースィング

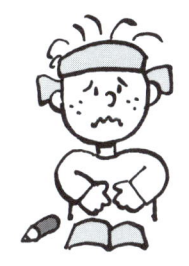

きりきりする痛み

soreness
ソーアーネス

（炎症などで）ひりひりする痛み

terrible pain
テリブル

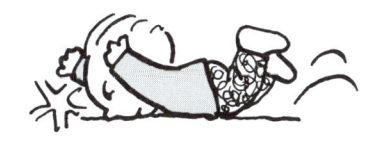

ひどい痛み

throbbing pain
スラビング

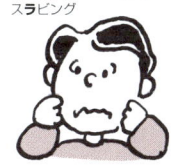

ずきずきする痛み

constant pain：絶え間ない痛み
カンスタントゥ

強い痛み：intense/severe pain
　　　　　インテンス　スィヴィア

COLUMN いろいろな痛み

痛みや苦痛を表す一般的な語はpain(ペィン)で，肉体的な痛みにも精神的な痛みにも用いられます．headacheやstomachacheで有名なache(エィク)は，身体の一部に起こる鈍痛のことです．

Lesson 8-A

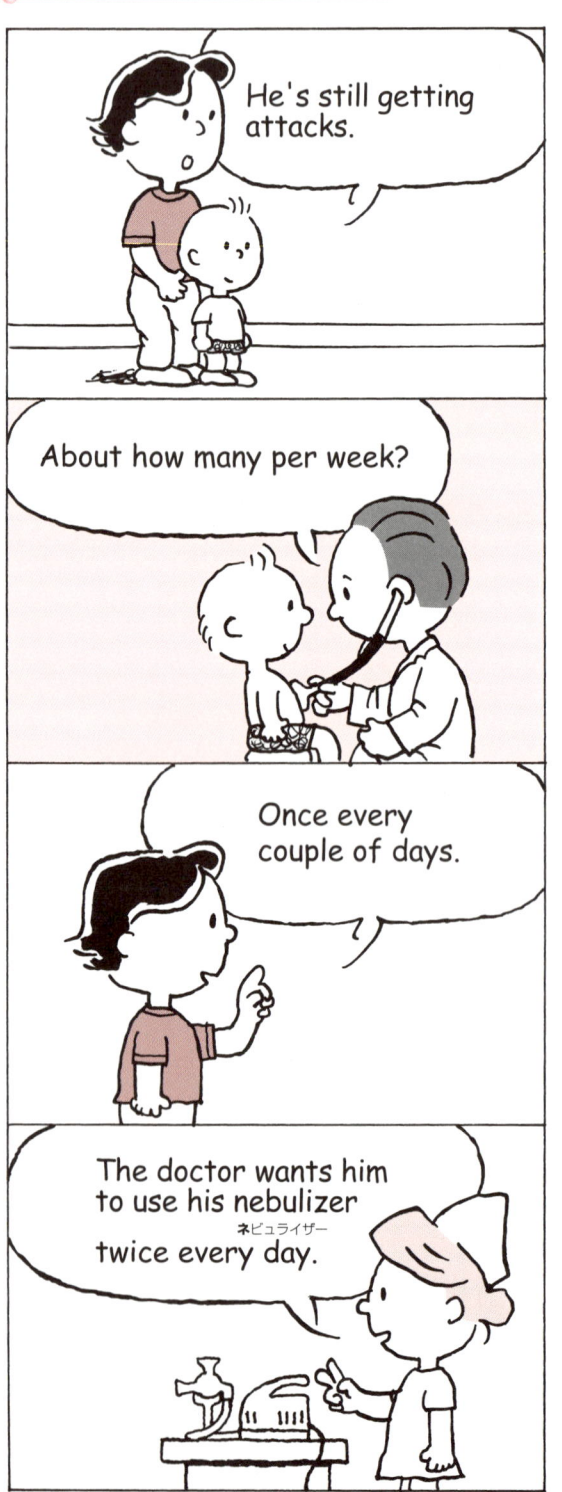

小児科―喘息

Pediatrics-Asthma

> He's still getting attacks.

M：まだ発作が起こります．

☞ 発作には，attack以外にseizureがある．attackは病気に使われる（例．heart attack）．seizure（スィージュアー）は，急激に症状が現われるてんかんに使われる．

> About how many per week?

D：週に何回くらいですか？

☞ How often do they occur? という尋ね方もある．

> Once every couple of days.

M：2日に1回くらいです．

> The doctor wants him to use his nebulizer (ネビュライザー) twice every day.

N：先生からの指示では，1日に2回ネブライザーで吸入してくださいということでした．

☞ nebulizerの代わりに，もっと小さく手で支えられるinhaler（インヘイラー）もある．

Vocabulary をふやそう

mumps
マムプス
おたふくかぜ

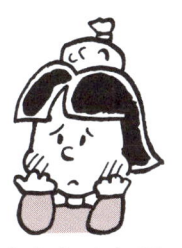

pertussis, whooping cough
パータスィス　フーピング　コフ
百日咳

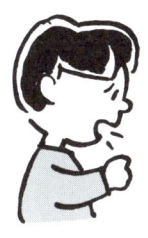

measles：はしか
ミーズルズ

rubella, German measles：風疹
ルベラ

chickenpox：水疱瘡
チキンパックス

diphtheria：ジフテリア
ディフスィリア

tetanus：破傷風
テタナス

encephalitis：脳炎
エンセファライティス

💡 予防接種（vaccination　ヴァクスィネイション）のMMRは，mumps, measles, rubellaのこと，DPT（いわゆる三種混合）は，diphtheria, pertussis, tetanusのこと．

子供に見られる症状や状態

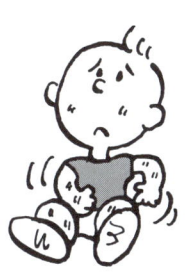

heat rash
あせも

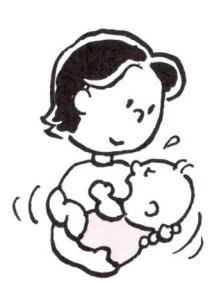

diaper rash：おむつかぶれ
ダイパー　ラッシュ

bronchitis：気管支炎
ブロンカイティス

tonsillitis：扁桃炎
タンシライティス

convulsion(s)：痙攣，ひきつけ
カンヴァルション

bed-wetting：夜尿症
ベッドゥウエッティング

31

Lesson 8-B

内科 — 摂食障害
Internal Medicine – Eating Disorders

My daughter is hardly eating and is so skinny.

M：この子，なかなか食べてくれなくて，こんなに痩せています．

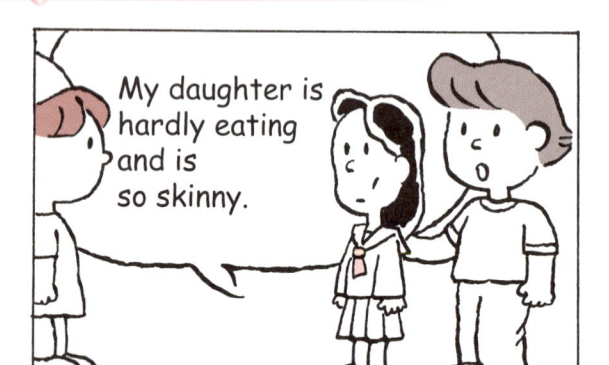

Are you dieting? Are your periods regular?

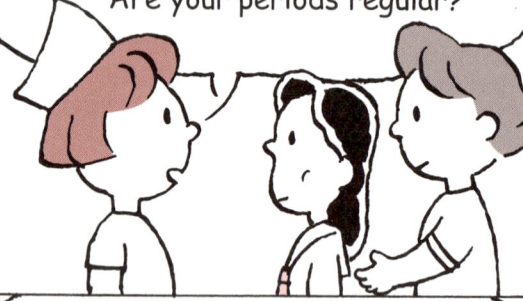

N：ダイエットしているの？ 生理はちゃんと来ているかしら？

☞ 生理(月経)は，正式には monthly period あるいは menstruation という．

Well, I have missed three periods... I just don't want to gain weight.

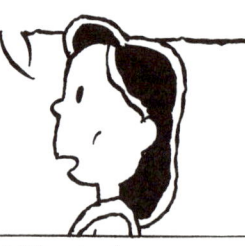

P：この3か月ほどは生理が来ていません…．体重が増えるのが嫌なんです．

I'd like to hear more about this. Let's talk in here while your mother waits for you in the waiting room.

N：そのことについて，もっとお聞きしたいので，お母さんに待合室で待ってもらっている間に，ここでもう少し話しましょう．

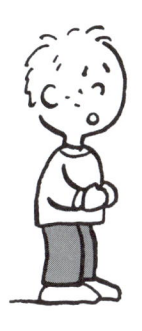

Vocabulary をふやそう

anorexia：拒食症
アノレクスィア

bulimia：過食症
ブリミア

anxiety：不安症
アングザイエティー

depression：うつ
ディプレッション

neurosis：神経症
ニューロウスィス

alcohol abuse：アルコール乱用
アルコホール アビューズ

drug addiction：薬物中毒
ドゥラッグ アディクション

violence：暴力行為
ヴァイオレンス

気持ちを訴える患者…なんて答えよう？？？

I'm depressed. / I'm feeling down.
ディプレストゥ
落ち込んでいます．

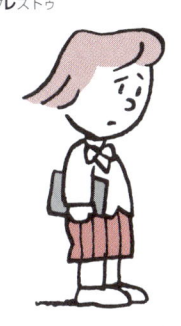

I'm worried about my work, and I can't sleep very well.
仕事のことが心配で
熟睡できません．

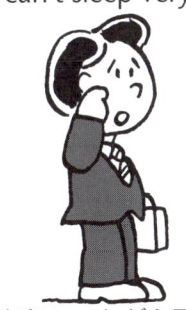

I'm nervous. / I have butterflies in my stomach.
緊張しています．

I don't have confidence in myself.
自分に自信がありません．

COLUMN 摂食障害とは？ Concerning Eating Disorders

摂食障害とは，10代の女子に多く見られる食行動の異常と，それに起因する無月経（amenorrhea）や激やせなどの症状を指し，神経性無食欲症（拒食症 anorexia）と神経性過食症（bulimia）に分かれます．ただし，多くの場合，両者は共存していて，神経性食欲不振症（anorexia nervosa）と呼ばれ，食べないだけでなく，一時的に過食状態になり嘔吐をくり返します．重度の場合は入院が必要ですが，カウンセリングやグループワーク，薬物療法，作業療法などの治療もあります．

Lesson 9-A

眼科—老人性白内障
Ophthalmology – Senile Cataracts

I can't see very well.

P：目がよく見えません．

I think you should consider cataract surgery.

D：白内障の手術を考えた方がいいですね．

Will I have to go to the hospital?

P：入院しなければなりませんか？

☞ admission も入院という意味．Do I need to be admitted? ともいう．

You may go home that day or stay in the hospital a day or two.

N：日帰りも可能ですし，入院しても1～2日です．

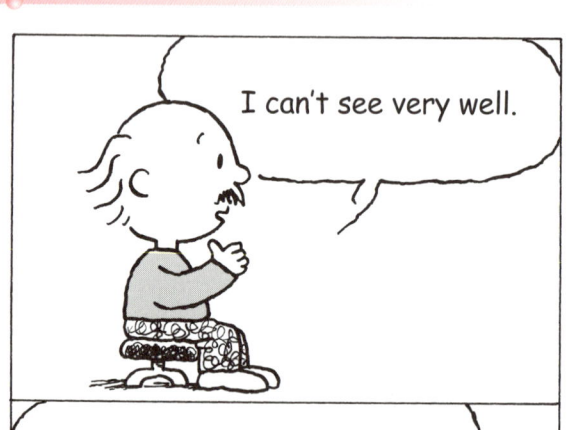

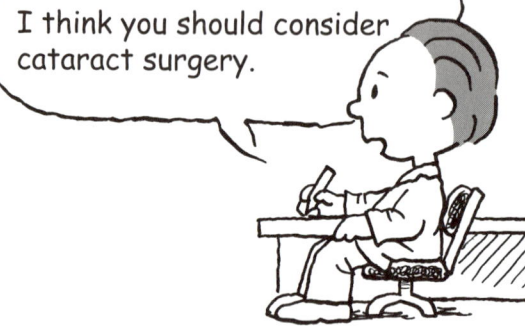

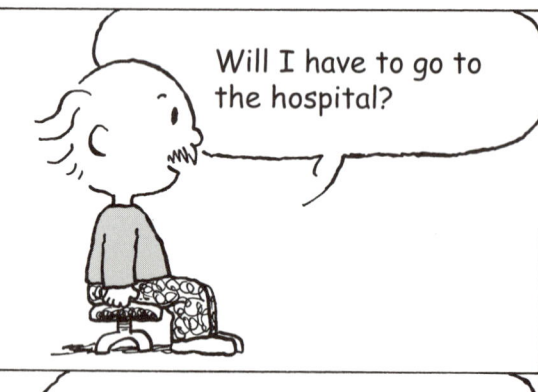

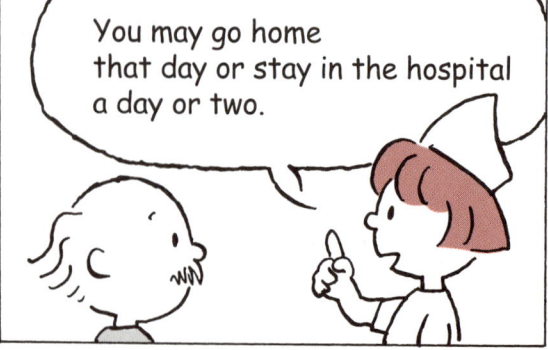

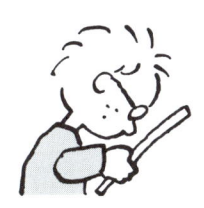

Vocabulary をふやそう

nearsightedness
ニア**サイ**ティドゥネス

近視

farsightedness
ファー**サイ**ティドゥネス

遠視

astigmatism：乱視
アス**ティ**グマティズム

intraocular lens：眼内レンズ
イントゥラ**ア**キュラー

macular degeneration：黄斑変性
マキュラー　ディジェネ**レイ**ション

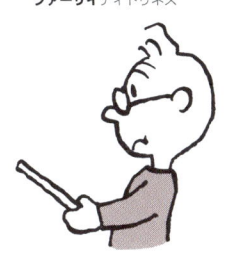

retinal detachment：網膜剥離
レティナル　ディ**タッ**チメントゥ

glaucoma：緑内障
グラウ**コウ**マ

laser treatment：レーザー治療
レイザー　トゥ**リー**トゥメントゥ

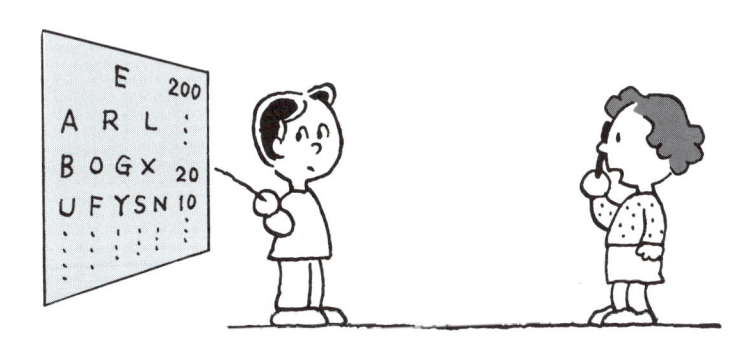

COLUMN 目の話　About Our Eyes

アメリカの視力検査は日本の方式と異なります．患者はチャートを20フィート（約6メートル）離れて読みます．正常な視力の人は20と書かれた横列が読めるはずで，その場合は20：20と呼ばれます．近視（nearsightedness, myopia）の人はそれより大きな文字しか読めないはずですから，20：30，20：40，20：50となります．20：30の意味は，正常な視力の人なら30フィートから読める文字を，その人は20フィートからしか読めないということです．逆に遠視（farsightedness, hyperopia）の人は20：10となり，その意味は正常な人が10フィートからしか見えない小さな文字を20フィートから読めるということです．なお，老眼という言葉は英語にありません．老眼は遠視ですので，**I've become farsighted.** と言います．そこで老眼鏡は，**reading glasses**と呼びます．

Lesson 9-B

耳鼻咽喉科 — 急性中耳炎 ENT-Acute Otitis Media

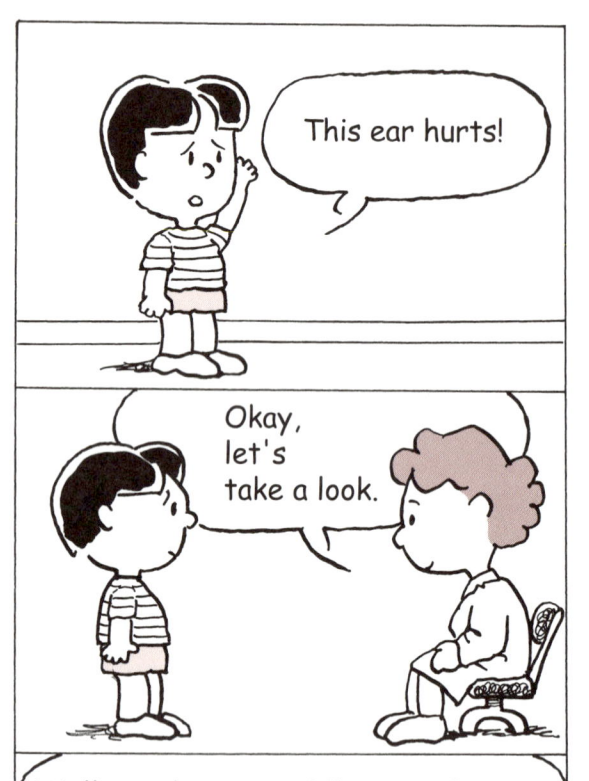

This ear hurts!

P：こっちの耳が痛いよ〜！

Okay, let's take a look.

D：どれ，見せてごらん．

Well, you have a middle ear infection. Maybe you got water in your ears at the pool?

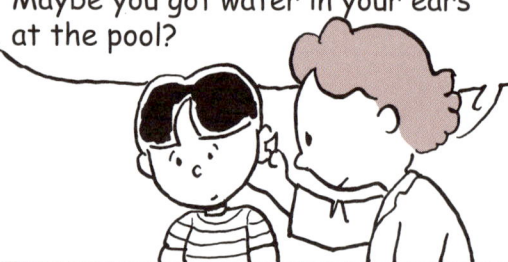

D：中耳炎になっちゃったね．たぶん，プールの水が耳に入ったのかな．

☞ 専門的には中耳炎のことを internal otitis (オウタイティス) あるいは otitis media という．

The doctor will give you a prescription for an antibiotic. Please take it to the pharmacy.

N：抗生物質の処方箋が出ますので，薬局へ持っていってね．

Vocabulary をふやそう

allergic rhinitis：アレルギー性鼻炎
アラージィク ライナイティス

hay fever：花粉症
ヘイ フィーヴァー

nosebleed：鼻出血
ノーズブリードゥ

eardrum：鼓膜
イアドゥラム

earache：耳痛
イアエイク

discharge：分泌物，排出物，退院
ディスチャージ

sore throat：咽頭痛
ソーアー スロウトゥ

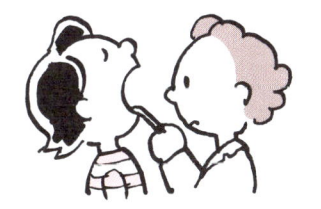

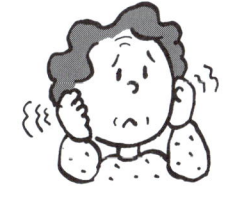

耳鼻咽喉科の症状を表現してみよう！

I get hoarse.
ホース

声が嗄(か)れます．

My grandfather has difficulty hearing.

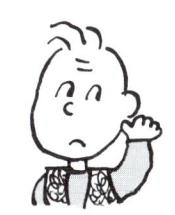

祖父は耳が聞こえにくいです．

Your symptoms probably
スィムプタムズ
come from cedar pollen.
スィーダー パレン

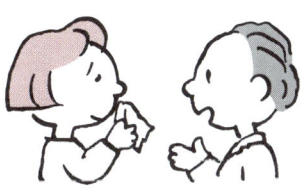

あなたの症状はおそらく
スギ花粉によるものでしょう．

You have swollen tonsils.
スウォルン タンスィルズ

扁桃腺が腫れていますよ．

I hear ringing or buzzing in my ears.
リンイング バズィング

耳鳴がします．

Lesson 10-A

皮膚科—アトピー性皮膚炎 Dermatology–Atopic Dermatitis

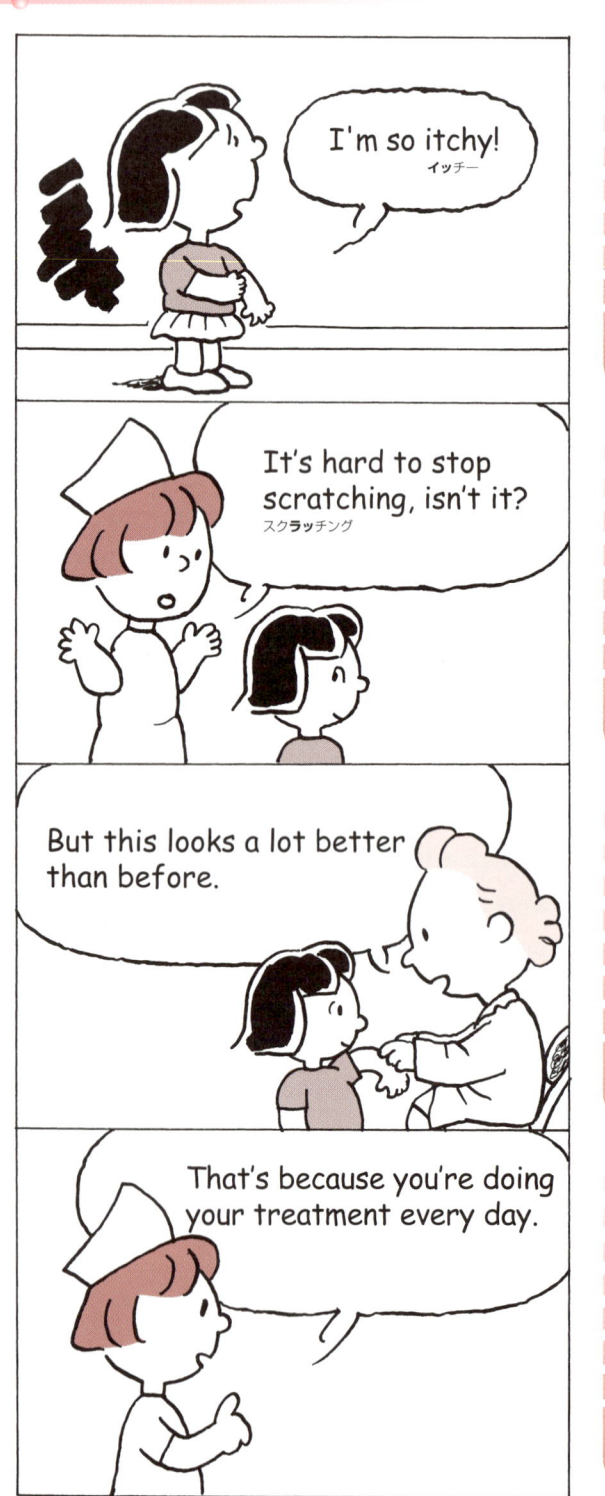

I'm so itchy!
イッチー

P：すごくかゆい．

It's hard to stop scratching, isn't it?
スクラッチング

N：掻き出すとやめられなくなっちゃうわよね？

But this looks a lot better than before.

D：でも，以前よりずっと良くなっているわよ．

That's because you're doing your treatment every day.

N：それは毎日自分で治療をがんばっているからよね．

📖 Vocabulary をふやそう

itching, pruritus
プルライタス

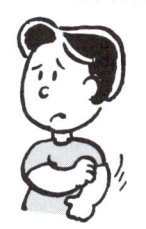

かゆみ，掻痒症

swelling, puffiness

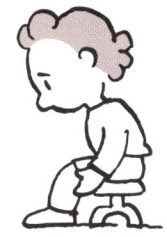

腫脹，むくみ

eczema：湿疹
エクゼマ

hives：じんま疹
ハイヴス

redness, erythema：紅斑
エリスィーマ

papules：丘疹
パピュルズ

erosion：ただれ
イロージョン

salve, ointment：軟膏
サーヴ　オイントゥメントゥ

steroids：ステロイド類
ステロイズ

bath treatment：入浴療法

皮膚の状態を英語にしてみよう！

cracked skin, chapped skin

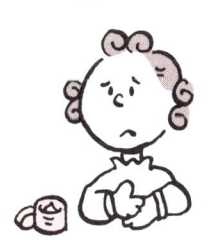

ひび割れの生じた肌

inflamed skin
インフレイムドゥ

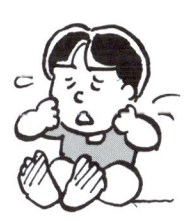

炎症を起こした肌

pimply skin

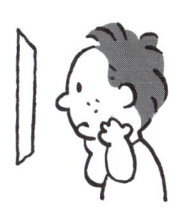

吹き出物だらけの肌

dry skin, desiccated skin：かさかさの肌
デスィケイティドゥ

oily skin：脂性の肌

irritated skin：荒れた肌
イリテイティドゥ

scarred skin：瘢痕（傷跡）肌
スカードゥ

Lesson 10-B

泌尿器科―前立腺肥大症 Urology–Prostatic Hypertrophy

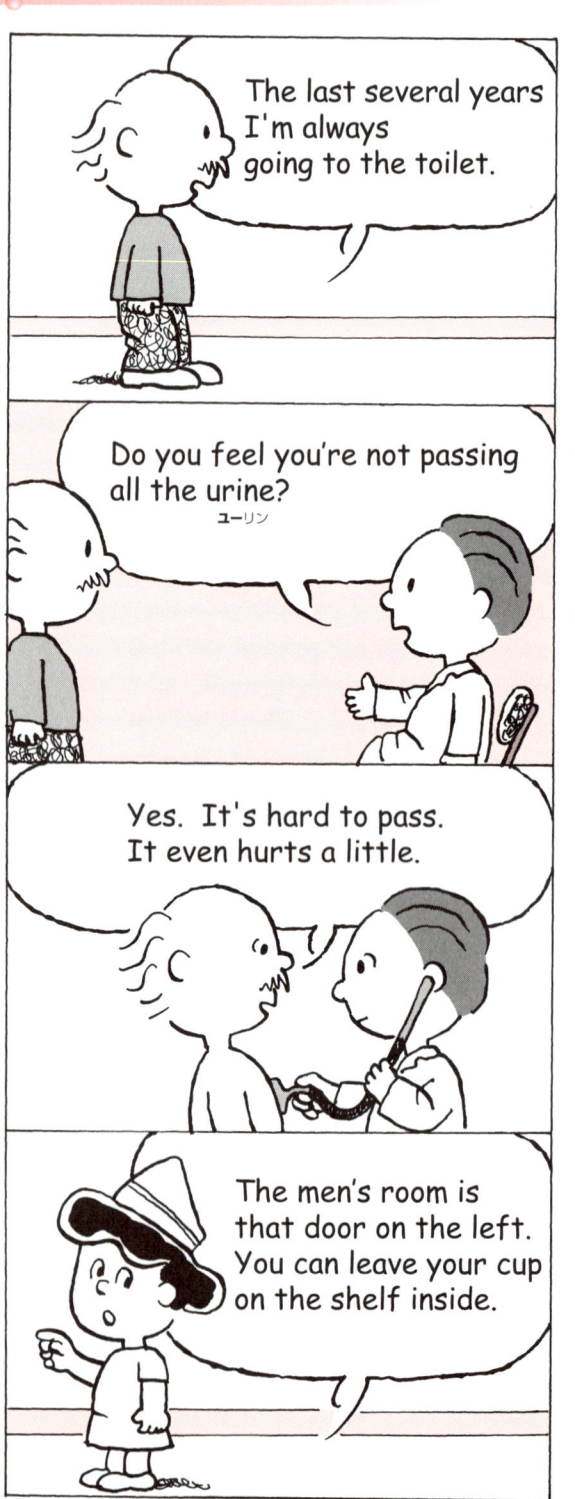

The last several years I'm always going to the toilet.

P：数年前からよくトイレへ行くようになりました．

Do you feel you're not passing all the urine?
ユーリン

D：尿を出し切れない感じですか？

☞ 日常会話では，urine の代わりに water を使う．

Yes. It's hard to pass. It even hurts a little.

P：はい．なかなか出ないし，少し痛いです．

The men's room is that door on the left. You can leave your cup on the shelf inside.

N：男性のトイレはあの左手のドアのところです．カップは中の棚の上に置いてください．

40

Vocabulary をふやそう

bladder：膀胱
ブラッダー

urinary frequency：頻尿
ユリナリー　フリークエンスィー

urinary retention：残尿
　　　　リテンション

ureteral calculus：尿管結石
ユリトゥラル　キャルキュラス

prostatectomy：前立腺切除術
プロスタテクトミー

Foley catheter：フォーリー・カテーテル
フォーリー　キャセター

sexual dysfunction：性的機能障害
　　　ディスファンクション

排泄の話

How many times per day do you urinate (have a bowel movement)?
ユリネイトゥ

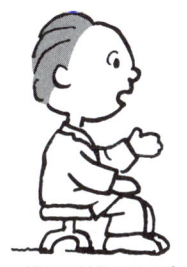

1日何回，排尿（排便）がありますか？

I have a heavy sensation in my stomach.

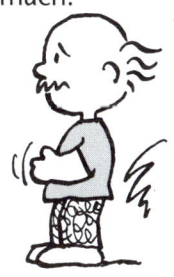

胃がもたれます．

My stomach makes rumbling sounds.
　　　　　　　　　ランブリング

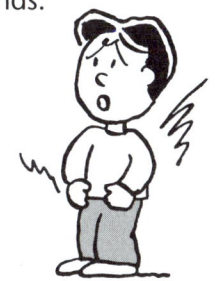

おなかがゴロゴロします．

I need to go.

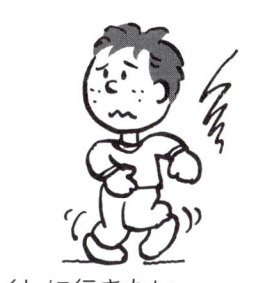

トイレに行きたい．

Do you feel that your bladder doesn't completely empty?
　　　　　　　　　　　ブラダー

　残尿感はありますか？

Do you feel a burning sensation with urination?

　排尿時に焼け付くような痛みがありますか？

There's a stone caught in your ureter. We need to decide on either an abdominal surgery or ESWL．
　　　　　　　　　　　　　　ユリター

　尿管に石がつまっています．開腹手術をするか，ESWL にするか決めなければなりません．

　（ESWL：extracorporeal shock wave lithotripsy　体外衝撃波結石破砕術）
　　　　　エクストゥラコーポリアル　　　　リソトゥリプスィー

Lesson 11-A

産科―妊娠　　Obstetrics－Pregnancy

The test shows that you're pregnant.
プレグナントゥ

D：検査結果によると，妊娠されていますね．

I feel so happy.
My husband and I have been hoping for a baby.

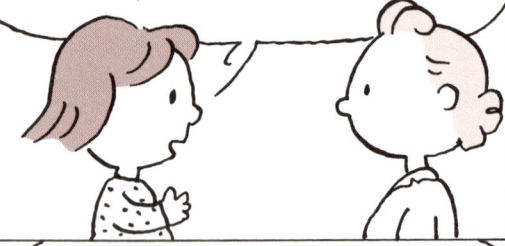

P：よかったわ．夫も私も赤ちゃんを望んでいましたから．

Your delivery date will be
デリヴァリー
about February 11th of next year.

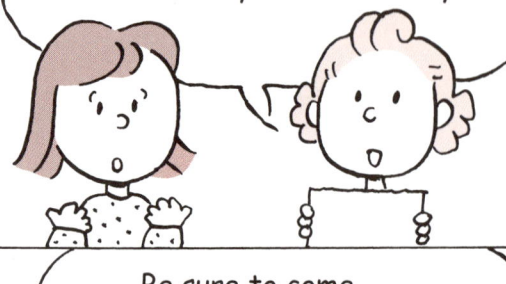

D：出産予定日は来年の2月11日ですよ．

Be sure to come for regular check-ups.
チェック アップス

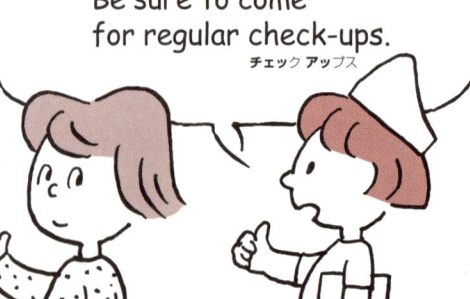

N：定期検査には必ず来てくださいね．

Vocabulary をふやそう

delivery：出産
デリヴァリー

fetus：胎児
フィータス

morning sickness：つわり
スィックネス

contraception, birth control：避妊
カントゥラセプション

abortion：妊娠中絶，流産
アボーション

period, menstruation：月経，生理
ピアリアッドゥ メンストゥルエイション

Lamaze method：ラマーズ法
ラマーズ

local anesthesia：局所麻酔
アネススィージア

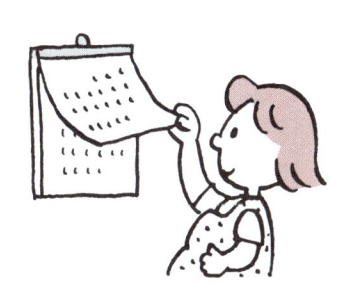

産科で使われる表現

I feel nauseated and have lost my appetite.
ノーズィエイティドゥ　　　　　アペタイトゥ
吐き気がして食欲がありません．

I missed my period.
ピアリアッドゥ
生理がありません．

My periods are regular (irregular).
月経は順調です(不順です)．

I had a cesarean section.
スィゼリアン
帝王切開をしました．

I had a miscarriage in my 4th week.
ミスキャリッジ
4週目で流産をしました．

COLUMN　HIV/AIDSの深刻な話　Some Serious Thoughts on HIV and AIDS

平成14年12月の統計によると，HIV感染者とAIDS患者の累計数は7,670名で，毎年10％強の割合で増加しています．HIV(ヒト免疫不全ウイルス；human immunodeficiency virus)は，リンパ球に感染し，免疫系を次々と破壊していくウイルスで，AIDS(後天性免疫不全症候群；acquired immune deficiency syndrome)はHIV感染が進み，肺炎(*Pneumocystis carinii*, pneumonia)などの合併症(complication)を引き起こした状態のことです．ただ，HIVに感染しても潜伏期間が長いため，すぐには発症せず，この期間はエイズ・キャリアと呼ばれます．治療法の進歩により発症を遅らせることができるようになってきましたが，死の恐怖を伴う疾患に変わりありません．HIVは感染者の血液(blood)，精液(sperm)，腟分泌液(secretion)に多く含まれ，母乳にも少し含まれます．感染経路は同性間性的接触(54%)，異性間性的接触(33%)，残りが輸血や事故などです．性感染が多いことから，性的接触時のコンドーム使用が重要であることがわかります．

Lesson 11-B

放射線科−X線治療 — Radiology Dept.−X-Ray Therapy

We'll need to do X-ray therapy.

D：X線治療を行わなければなりません．

☞ radiation therapy（レイディエイション セラピー）ともいう．

How long will that take?

P：どのくらい行うのですか？

Once or twice a day for five days a week, continuing for six to seven weeks.

D：1日1〜2回，週5日を，6〜7週間続けます．

Maybe that sounds like a lot, but let's work together to get you well.

N：大変なように聞こえるかもしれませんが，治るように一緒にがんばりましょう．

Vocabulary をふやそう

X-ray films：X線フィルム，レントゲン写真
エックスレイ

side effects：副作用
イフェクツ

leukopenia：白血球減少症
ルコピニア

radiation burns：放射線熱傷
バーンズ

brain tumor：脳腫瘍
トゥーマー

PET (positron emission tomography) scan：PETスキャン
パズィトゥロン　イミッション　トマグラフィー　スキャン

治療や病気，検査について患者はわかっているかしら？

Did your doctor inform you about your therapy (your disease, the result of the test)?

Have you read the consent form?
カンセントゥ

Is there anything you want to ask the doctor or the nurse?

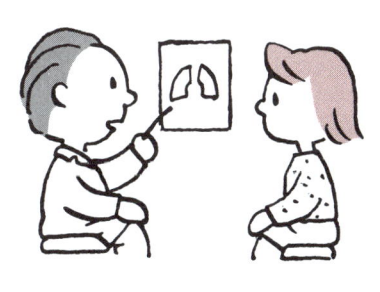

担当医から治療（病気，検査結果）について説明がありましたか？

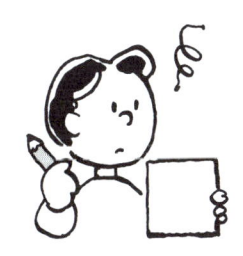

承諾書を読みましたか？

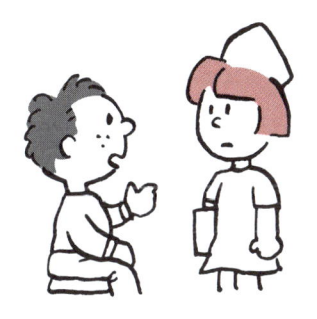

医師や看護師に尋ねたいことはありますか？

Could you understand what your doctor said?
　担当医が話した内容を理解できましたか？

Are you satisfied with the doctor's explanation?
　医師の説明に納得されましたか？

Lesson 12-A

歯科—虫歯

Dentistry-Cavities

Open your mouth wide.

DE：あ〜んと口を開けて．

Uh oh, here's a cavity.
キャヴィティー

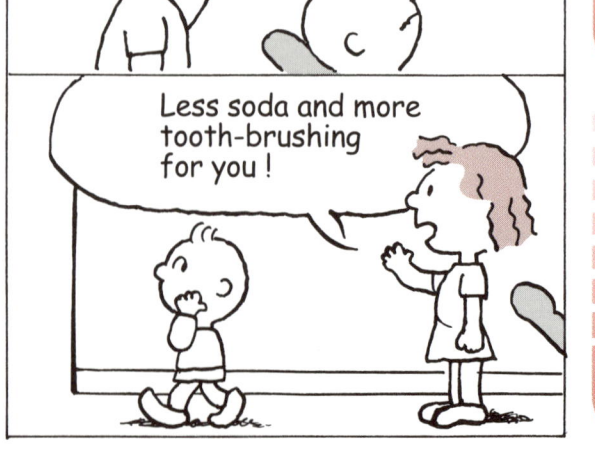

DE：あっ，ここに虫歯があるわ．

The dentist can fix that so it won't hurt.

DH：先生が痛まないように治してくれますよ．

Less soda and more tooth-brushing for you!

DH：ソーダを控えて，もっと歯磨きをしてね．

Vocabulary をふやそう

cavity, dental caries,
キャーリーズ
decayed tooth
ディケイドゥ

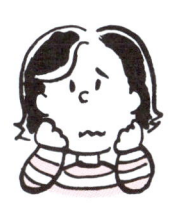

虫歯

denture
デンチャー

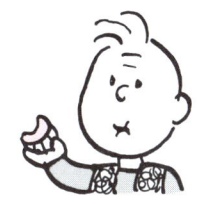

義歯・入れ歯

toothache：歯痛
トゥースエイク

molar：大臼歯
モウラー

wisdom tooth：親知らず
ウィズダム

root canal：根管
カナル

filling：充填

crown：歯冠

bridge：ブリッジ

歯科で聞かれるフレーズを覚えよう！

Brush your teeth before going to bed.
　寝る前に歯をよく磨きましょう．

It's better to drink tea than carbonated drinks / soda.
　　　　　　　　　　　　　　　カーボネイティドゥ
　炭酸水／ソーダではなくお茶を飲むほうがいいですよ．

It's helpful to use a fluoride toothpaste.
　　　　　　　　　フルオライドゥ　トゥースペイストゥ
　フッ素入り歯磨剤を使ったほうがいいですよ．

COLUMN 耳よりな歯のはなし　How Cavities Form

虫歯（caries）はS.ミュータンス菌が歯に付着して，表面を溶かすことにより生じます．従来，甘いものや炭酸飲料水を控えるよう指導がされていましたが，現在では少し違う指導が考えられています．甘いものも炭酸飲料水も食事中や食後にとれば，唾液（saliva）の分泌が促されているため，あまり問題はありません．この唾液が歯の表面を守り，虫歯になりにくくするからです．一方，虫歯を誘発するのは，食間に甘いものや炭酸飲料水を口にすることです．就寝前の正しい歯磨きと，できれば食後の歯磨きを励行し，間食しないことが大切です．

Lesson 12-B

歯科─歯肉炎

Dentistry-Gingivitis

In the back on the right there's a place that bleeds.

There's some pyorrhea there.
パイオリーア

Can that be cured?

With proper brushing, it should improve quite a lot.

P：右奥から出血があります．

DE：そこは歯槽膿漏になっていますね．

P：治りますか？

DH：正しいブラッシングをすれば，かなりよくなりますよ．

Vocabulary をふやそう

bleeding：出血
ブリーディング

drainage：排膿
ドゥレイネッジ

tartar：歯石
ターター

breath odor, halitosis：口臭
ブレス　　オウダー　　ハリトウスィス

gum recession：歯肉退縮

dental hygienist：歯科衛生士
デンタル　　ハイジェニストゥ

dental implant：歯のインプラント
　　　　イムプラントゥ

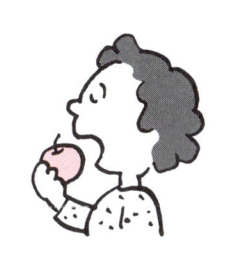

歯の状態を表現してみよう！

There's stabbing pain, when I drink cold water.

冷たい水を飲むとしみます．

My gums bleed when I brush.

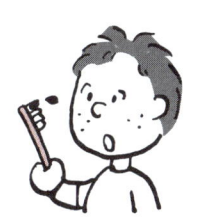

歯を磨くと出血します．

I have a loose tooth.

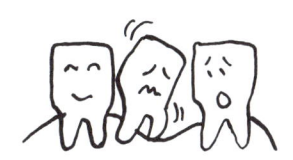

グラグラする歯があります．

I need my teeth straightened. / I need orthodontics.
　　　　　　　　　　オーソドンティクス

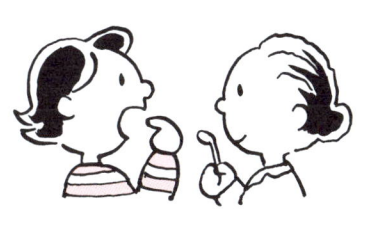

歯の矯正をしたいです．

Lesson 13-A

救命救急室—交通事故　Emergency Room – Traffic Accident

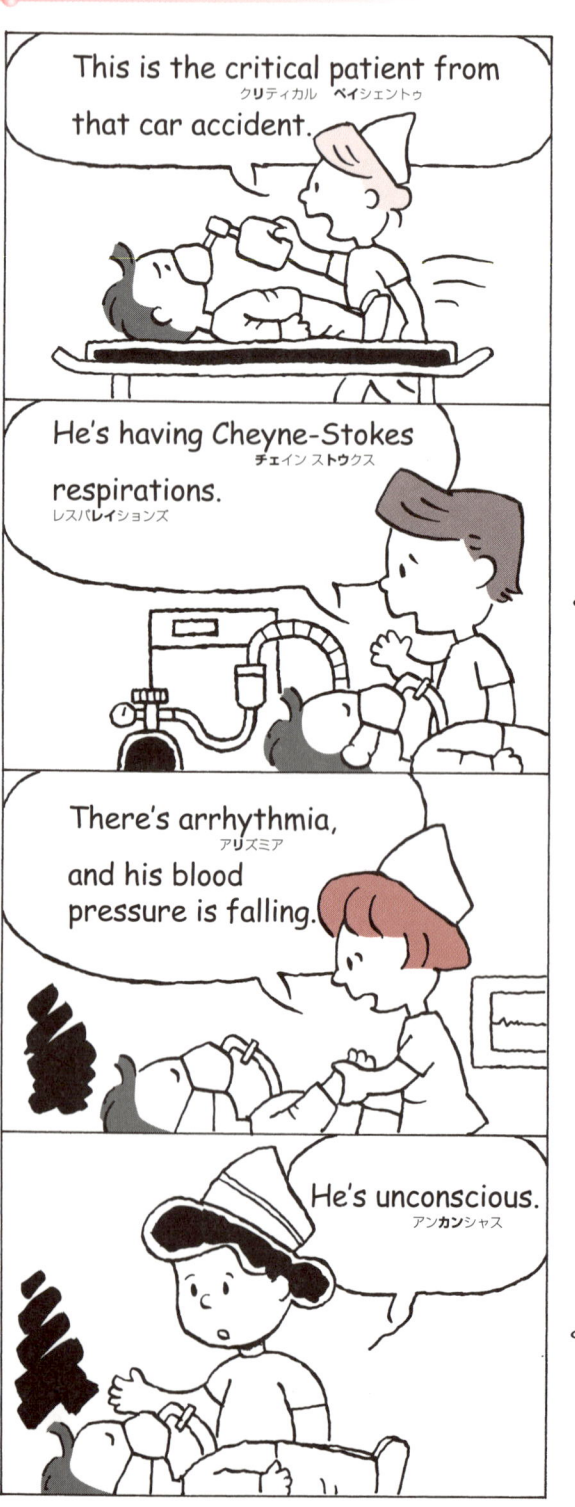

This is the critical patient from that car accident.

N1：交通事故の急患です．

He's having Cheyne-Stokes respirations.

N2：呼吸はチェーンストークス．

☞ チェーンストークスとは，無呼吸と過換気を交互に繰り返す状態のこと．

There's arrhythmia, and his blood pressure is falling.

N3：不整脈があり，血圧が下がってきています．

He's unconscious.

N4：意識はありません．

☞ He's lost consciousness.と言い換えることもできる．in comaで昏睡状態の意．

Vocabulary をふやそう

trauma：外傷
トゥローマ

lifesaving equipment, "crash cart"：
イグイップメントゥ　　緊急用(医療処置)カート

resuscitation：蘇生
リサスィテイション

complete blood count (CBC)：全血球計算，全血算

transfusion：輸血
トゥランスフュージョン

triage：トリアージ
トゥリアージュ
💡 患者の治療優先順位を決めること．

paramedic：救急救命士
パラメディク

救急でよく使われる表現1

My son is bleeding.

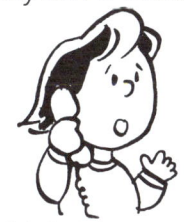

息子が出血を起こしています．

You've broken your femur.
フィーマー

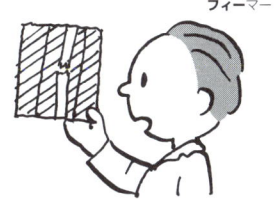

大腿骨を骨折しています．

She is critically ill. / She is severely injured.
彼女は重症です(重体です)．

There are signs that your father has
a brain hemorrhage.
ヘモレッジ
お父様には脳内出血の徴候が見られます．

I will check his vital signs.
バイタルサインを調べてみます．
💡 バイタルサインは，呼吸，脈拍，
血圧維持などを含む．

COLUMN 息子の臓器提供を励行したある夫妻の話
Fulfilling a Son's Desire to Donate Organs

筆者の知人に30歳の子息を亡くされた夫妻がいます．運動をした直後，クモ膜下出血で突然倒れた彼は，生前ドナーとして厚生省(現厚生労働省)の(社)日本臓器移植ネットワークに登録していました．そこで，彼の角膜，腎臓，組織，皮膚がそれぞれ別の患者に移植されました．腎臓をもらった女の子に，スプーン1杯のおしっこが出たとき，彼女の母親はとても喜んだそうです．自分の息子が臓器提供者になった母親が，今の気持ちを語ってくれました．「息子の葬儀のときに腎臓移植成功の朗報が届いたのですが，とても嬉しかったことを覚えています．焼き場で息子の遺骨が帰ってきたとき，不思議と喪失感はなく，体は生きている…と思いました．そして今でも…」

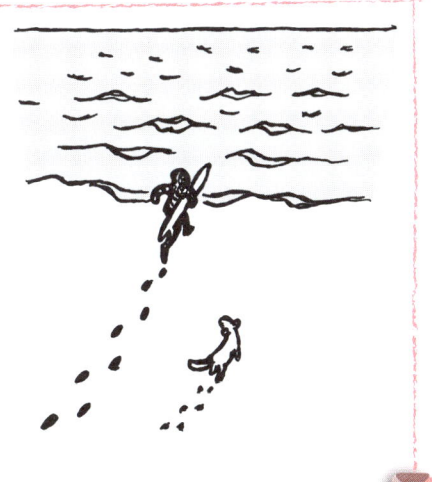

Lesson 13-B

救急―心肺蘇生法

Ambulance Call
―Cardiopulmonary Resuscitation

He has *mochi* caught in his throat!

FM：お餅が喉につかえた！

His dentures have slipped, too…

AA：入れ歯がはずれている….

I can't quite get it.

AA：取れそうで取れないよ．

There! The Heimlich maneuver got it out.

AA：やった！ハイムリック法で取れましたよ．

☞ ハイムリック法とは，食べ物などを喉につまらせた人の後ろから両腕でお腹を抱きかかえ，前に組んだ手でお腹から胸に向かって押し上げる救命法のこと．

Vocabulary をふやそう

airway obstruction：気道閉塞
アブストラクション

cyanosis：チアノーゼ
サイアノウスィス

oxygen：酸素
アクスジュン

oximeter, "pulse ox"：パルスオキシメーター
アクシミター　　　パルス　アックス

artificial respiration：人工呼吸
　　　　　レスパレイション

cardiac massage：心臓マッサージ
カーディアック マサージ

respiratory arrest：呼吸停止
レスパラトリー　　　アレスト

cardiac arrest：心停止
カーディアック アレストゥ

defibrillation：細動除去
ディフィブリレイション

ambulance attendant：救急隊員
アムビュランス　　アテンダントゥ

救急でよく使われる表現2

pulse
パルス
（carotid, brachial, radial）
　カラティドゥ　ブレイキアル　レイディアル
（regular, irregular,
　　　　　　イレギュラー
bradycardia, tachycardia）
ブレディーカーディア　タキーカーディア

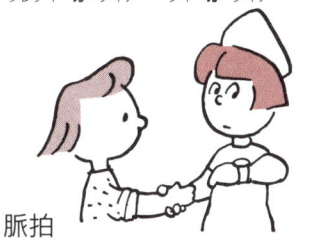

trauma
トゥローマ
（bleeding, cut,
scratch, bruise）
　　　　　ブルーズ

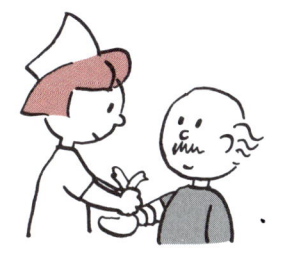

pupil response
（constriction, dilation）
カンストゥリクション　ダイレイション

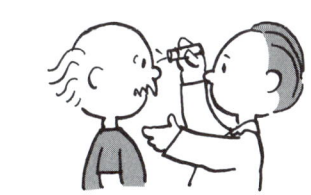

脈拍
（頸動脈，上腕動脈，橈骨動脈）
（整脈，不整脈，徐脈，頻脈）

外傷
（出血，切り傷，
擦過傷，打撲傷）

瞳孔反射（縮瞳，拡張）

temperature（axillary, oral, rectal）：体温（腋窩，口腔内，直腸）
テムパラチャー　　　アクシレリー　　オーラル　レクタル

blood pressure（systolic/diastolic）：血圧（収縮期/拡張期）
ブラッドゥ　　　　　スィスタリック ダイアスタリック

respiration（tachypnea, hyperventilation, bradypnea, shallow breathing）
レスパレイション　　タキプニア　　ハイパーヴェンティレイション　ブラディプニア
　　　　　　　　　　　　　　　　　　　　　　　：呼吸（頻呼吸，過換気，徐呼吸，浅い呼吸）

consciousness（conscious/comatose）：意識（意識のある/昏睡）
カンシャスネス　　　　　　　　　　コマトウス

COLUMN いろいろな傷

trauma（トゥローマ）は，"トラウマ"と日本語でも使われ，主として精神面でのダメージという意味ですが，医療では一般的に外傷のことを言います．事故での傷やけがは injury，武器による傷やけがは wound，軽いけがは hurt を使います．また，引っかいてできた傷は scratch ですが，擦れてできた傷は scrape と言います．

Lesson 14-A

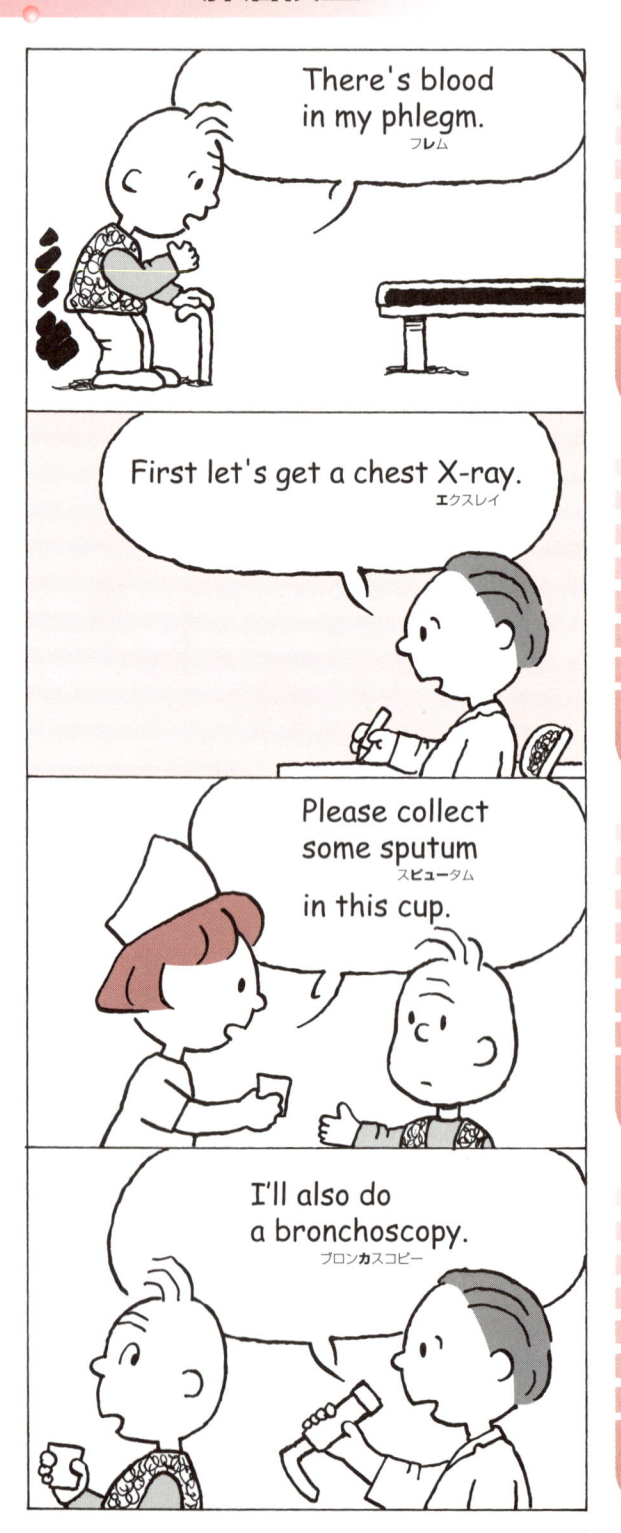

肺癌検査 / Lung Cancer Screening

There's blood in my phlegm.
フレム

P：痰に血が混じります．

First let's get a chest X-ray.
エクスレイ

D：まず胸部X線を撮りましょう．

Please collect some sputum in this cup.
スピュータム

N：このカップに痰を出してください．

I'll also do a bronchoscopy.
ブロンカスコピー

D：さらに，気管支鏡検査を行いますね．

Vocabulary をふやそう

asymptomatic, symptom-free：無症状
エイスィムプト**マ**ティック　ス**ィ**ムプタムフ**リ**ー

dyspnea, difficulty breathing：呼吸困難
ディスプニア

pneumothorax, collapsed lung：気胸
ニューモ**ソ**ラックス　コ**ラ**プストゥ

drain：ドレーン
ドゥ**レ**イン

tuberculosis (TB)：肺結核
トゥバキュ**ロ**ウスィス

remission：緩解
リ**ミ**ッション　　かんかい

relapse, recurrence：再発
リ**ラ**プス　リ**カ**レンス

MRI (magnetic resonance imaging)：
マグ**ネ**ティック　**レ**ゾナンス　**イ**メジィング
核磁気共鳴映像装置

CT (computed tomography)：
コン**ピュ**ーティドゥ　ト**マ**グラフィー
コンピュータ断層撮影装置

X線検査での指示

Undress from the waist up, please.
上半身だけ脱いでください．

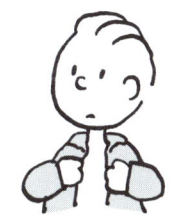

Take a deep breath and hold it. ブレス
深く息を吸ってから止めてください．

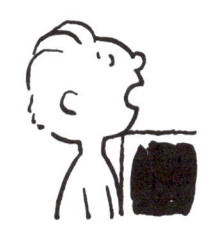

Lift your right arm.
右腕を上げてください．

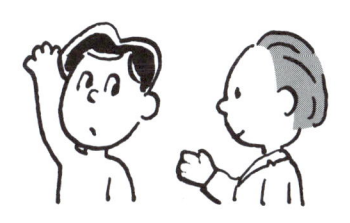

Please take off your watch and jewelry.
時計やアクセサリーを外してください

Turn to the right (left).
右（左）に向いてください．

COLUMN 乳癌の早期発見と乳房温存手術　Early Detection and Conservative Treatment of Breast Cancer

（1）自己検診（self-examination）を行う．
（2）乳房X線撮影検査（mammography）を受ける．
（3）超音波検査（echo, ultrasonography）を受ける．
（4）セカンド・オピニオン，サード・オピニオンを積極的に受ける．

乳房の全摘術（mastectomy）は，その後の心理的影響を考えると慎重にするべきです．初期であったり，患部が小さければ，乳房温存手術（breast conservation therapy）が考えられます．ただし，この場合，乳癌（breast cancer）の育つ母地となる乳腺（mammary gland）や，乳腺に散った癌細胞（cancer cell）が残っている可能性があり，再発（recurrence）の危険があります．そのため，乳房温存法の場合，術後に放射線治療（X-ray therapy）を行います．週5回で5週間が基準で，この放射線治療を併用すれば，再発の危険性が全摘とほぼ同程度になります．

Lesson 14-B

乳癌検査 / Breast Cancer Screening

I can feel a lump here in my left breast.

P：左胸にしこりがあるように感じます．

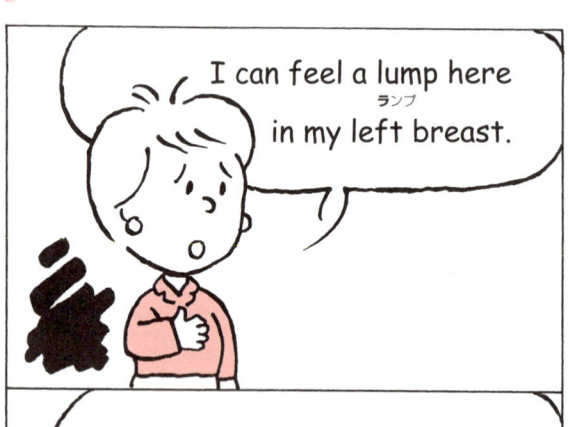

I can't be sure by palpation alone. Let's get some tests.

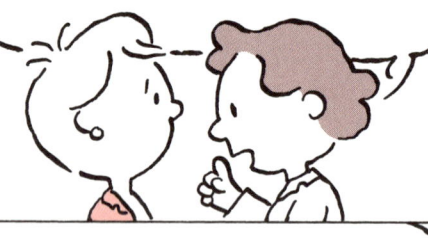

D：触診だけではわかりませんので，検査をしましょう．

(After the test) Your three test results do suggest cancer, but I think we've caught it early.

（検査後）
D：3つの検査の結果，悪性腫瘍だろうということがわかりましたが，早期発見のようでした．

☞ 3つの検査とは，マンモグラフィー，穿刺吸引細胞診，乳腺腫瘤摘出のこと．

It will be cured completely with the surgery, won't it?

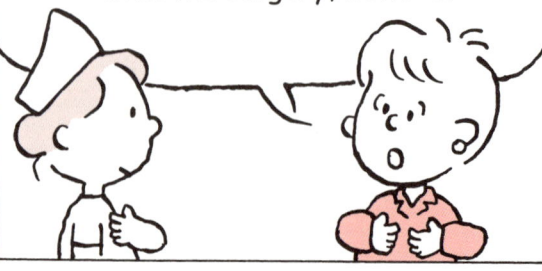

P：手術をすれば完治しますよね？

☞ 乳房切除は mastectomy という．

📖 Vocabulary をふやそう

mammography：マンモグラフィー
マモグラフィー

lumpectomy：乳腺腫瘤摘出
ランペクトミー

needle biopsy and cytodiagnosis：穿刺吸引細胞診
バイオプスィー　　　サイトダイアグノウスィス

benign tumor：良性腫瘍
ビナイン　トゥーマー

malignant tumor：悪性腫瘍
マリグナントゥ

chemotherapy：化学療法
キモセラピー

mastectomy：乳房切除
マステクトミー

prosthesis：プロテーゼ
プラススィースィス

lymph gland：リンパ腺
リンフ　グランドゥ

metastasis：転移
メタスタスィス

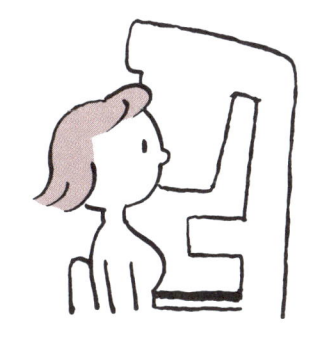

🚩 婦人科で使われる表現 🚩

Have you ever been pregnant?
／How many times
have you been pregnant?

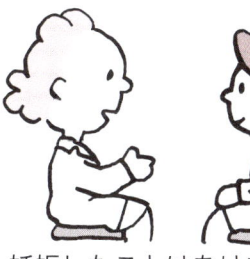

妊娠したことはありますか？
／何回妊娠しましたか？

Do you use
oral contraceptives
or hormone pills?

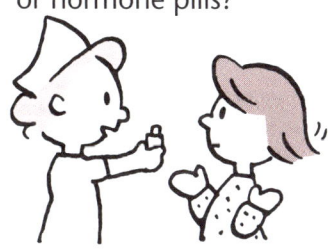

経口避妊薬やホルモン剤を
使っていますか？

I have hot flashes
in my face.　フラシィズ

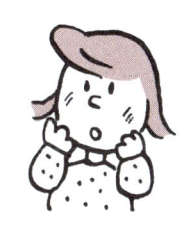

顔がのぼせます．

How often do your periods come?
　月経の周期はどれくらいですか？

Do you get (menstrual) cramps?
　生理痛がありますか？

I have a discharge.
　おりものがあります．

I have slight pain and bloating with my periods.
　　　　　　　　　　　　ブロウティング
　月経時に少し痛くなったり，（水分が保持され）体がむくみます．

Lesson 15-A

心臓検査—ホルター心電図　Cardiac Exam—Holter Monitor

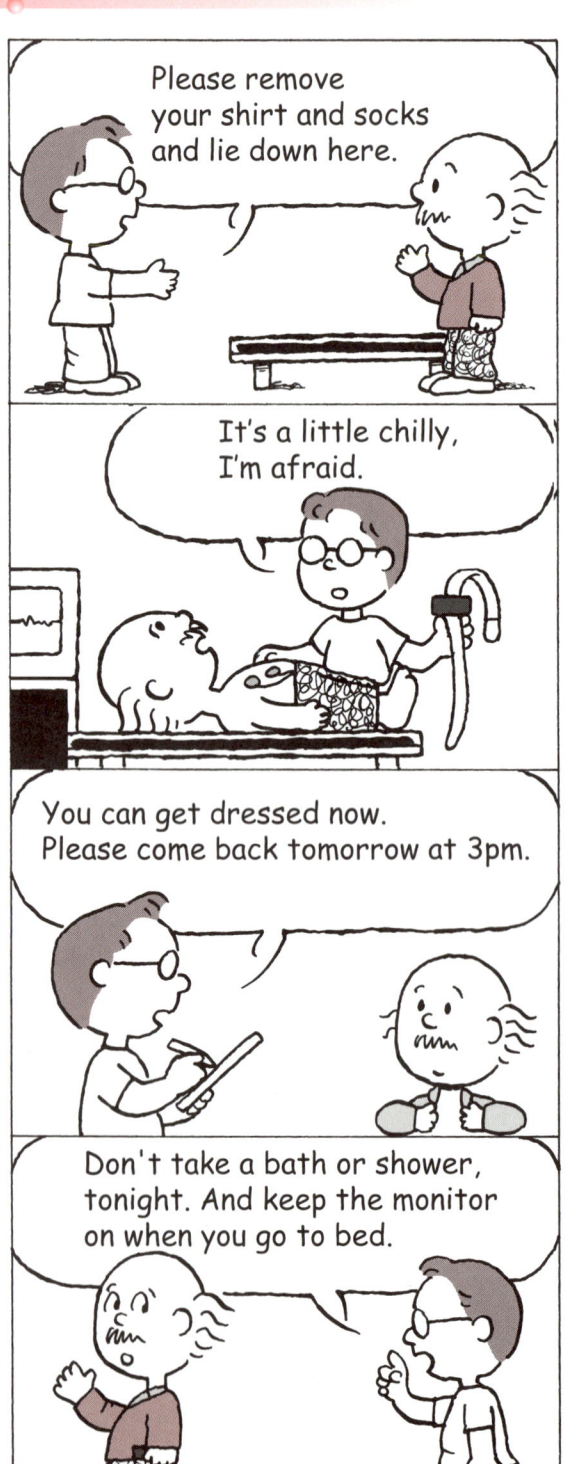

Please remove your shirt and socks and lie down here.

T：シャツと靴下を脱いで，ここに横になって下さい．

It's a little chilly, I'm afraid.

T：ちょっと冷たいですよ．

You can get dressed now. Please come back tomorrow at 3pm.

T：洋服を着てください．明日，午後3時にまた来てください．

Don't take a bath or shower, tonight. And keep the monitor on when you go to bed.

T：今夜はお風呂やシャワーに入らないでくださいね．モニターをそのままにして寝てください．

Vocabulary をふやそう

chest pain：胸痛

angina：狭心症
アンジナ

arrhythmia：不整脈
アリズミア

heart murmur：心雑音
マーマー

congestive heart failure：うっ血性心不全
カンジェスティヴ

heart attack：心臓発作

cardiac catheterization：心カテーテル検査
カーディアック キャセテリゼイション

salt restriction：塩分制限
ソルトゥ リストゥリクション

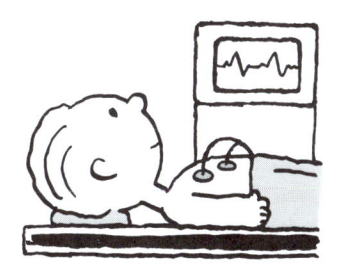

検査についての説明をしてみよう！

On the day of your test, go to the exam room reception desk and submit this appointment form.

Don't wear tight clothes on the day of your test.

You have to change to a hospital gown before the test.

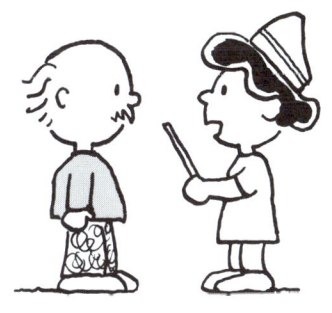

当日は検査室の窓口へ行き，この予約票をご提示ください．

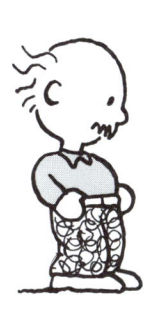

検査当日は締め付けるような服装を避けてください．

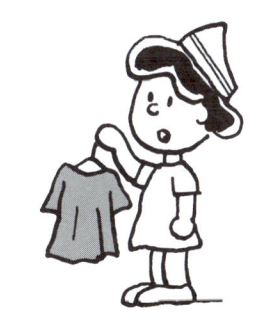

検査では検査用のガウンに着替えてもらいます．

Do not eat or drink anything except water after 9 pm the day before your test.
　　検査の前日は午後9時以降，水分以外は食べたり飲んだりしないでください．

You can't eat for 2 hours after this test.
　　検査後2時間は食事ができません．

Lesson 15-B

大腸検査　　Colonoscopy

Over the next hour, drink half of this liquid one-third every 20 minutes.

N：今から1時間をかけて，このボトルの液体半分を，20分ごとに3回に分けて飲んでください．

It will make you want to use the toilet over and over. That will clean out the bowel.

N：トイレに何度も何度も行きたくなります．それで腸がきれいになります．

Drink the other half of the liquid the same way, one-third every 20 minutes.

N：残り半分の液体を同様に，20分ごとに1時間かけ，3回に分けて飲んでください．

(Two hours later, at the laboratory)
Lie down on your side with your back toward me. Bend your upper leg a little.

（2時間後，検査室にて）
D：ベッドの上で横になり，こちらに背中を向ける形で横向きになってください．足を軽く曲げてください．

📖✏️ Vocabulary をふやそう

sedation：鎮静
セデイション

polyp：ポリープ
パリプ

hemorrhoids：痔
ヘモロイズ

bloody stools：血便
ストゥールズ

diarrhea：下痢
ダイアリア

constipation：便秘
カンスティペイション

colic, abdominal pain：疝痛
カリック　アブダミナル

intestinal obstruction：腸閉塞
インテスティナル　アブストゥラクション

🚩 検査中の患者への声かけ 🚩

This test will take about 30 minutes.

Please push this button if you have any pain or you feel sick.

Well done! It's over and you don't have to be nervous any more.

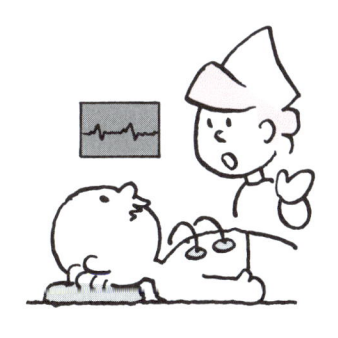

この検査は30分ほどかかります．

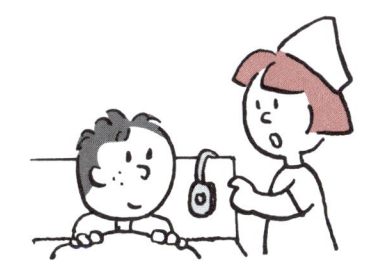

痛みがあったり気分が悪くなりましたら，このボタンを押してください．

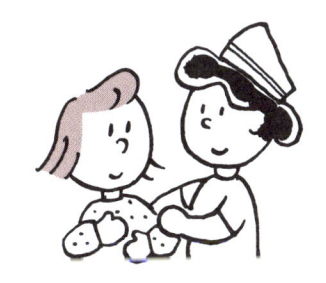

よくがんばりましたね．終わりましたから，もう緊張しなくてもいいですよ．

Be relaxed. I'll stay by your side.
　力を抜いてくださいね．私がそばにいますよ．

It will be finished in five more minutes. / It will be over soon.
　あと５分で終わりますよ．／もうすぐ終わりますよ．

Lesson 16-A

入院手続き

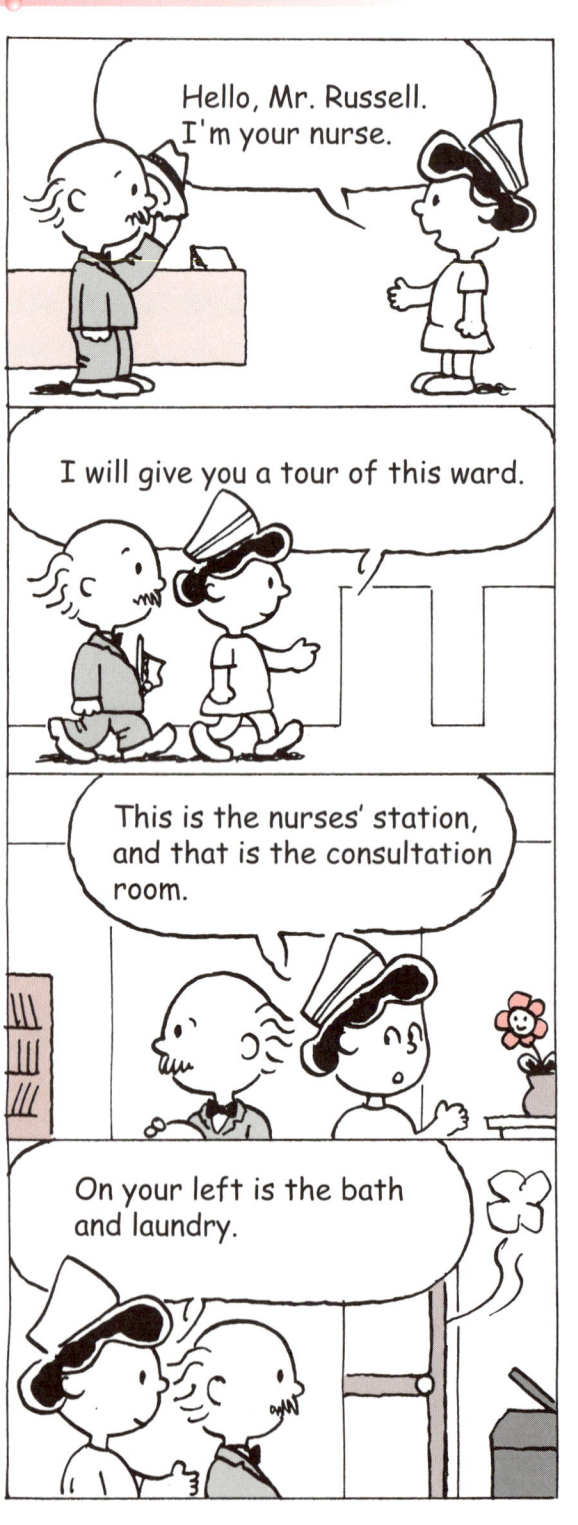

Admission

Hello, Mr. Russell. I'm your nurse.

N：こんにちは，ラッセルさん．私は担当の看護師です．

I will give you a tour of this ward.

N：この病棟の案内をしましょう．

This is the nurses' station, and that is the consultation room.

N：こちらがナースステーションで，あちらが相談室です．

On your left is the bath and laundry.

N：左側が浴室と洗濯場になっています．

Vocabulary をふやそう

reservation：予約
レザヴェイション

nurses' station：看護ステーション

food cart：配膳車

shower room：シャワー室

toilet, bathroom：トイレ

store, shop：売店

visitors' room：面会室

private room：個室

four-bed ward：四人部屋

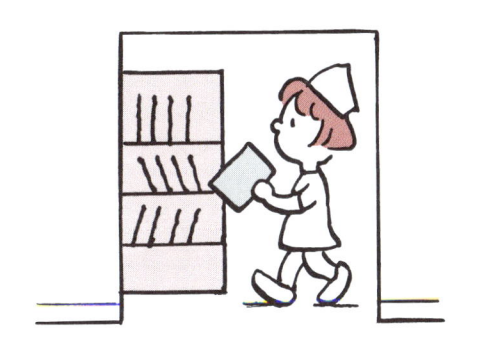

病院内を案内してみよう！

Take the elevator to the first floor and go right.
You will find the cafeteria.

Go straight down this corridor and turn left. You will see the sign for the X-ray lab.

The dining room is on the seventh floor. The scenery is beautiful from there.

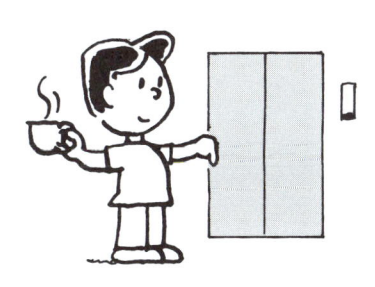

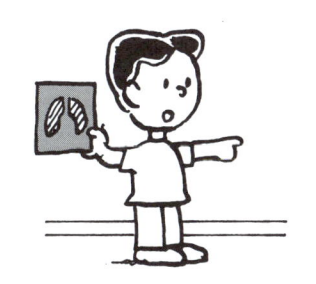

エレベータで1階まで行き，右へ行ってください．喫茶室があります．

この廊下をまっすぐ行って左に曲がってください．X線検査室のサインが見えるはずです．

食堂は7階にあります．そこからの眺めはいいですよ．

Mr. Tanaka's room is across from the nurses' station.
　　田中さんの病室はナースステーションの向かい側です．

The examination room is next to the consultation room.
　　診察室は相談室の隣です．

Lesson 16-B

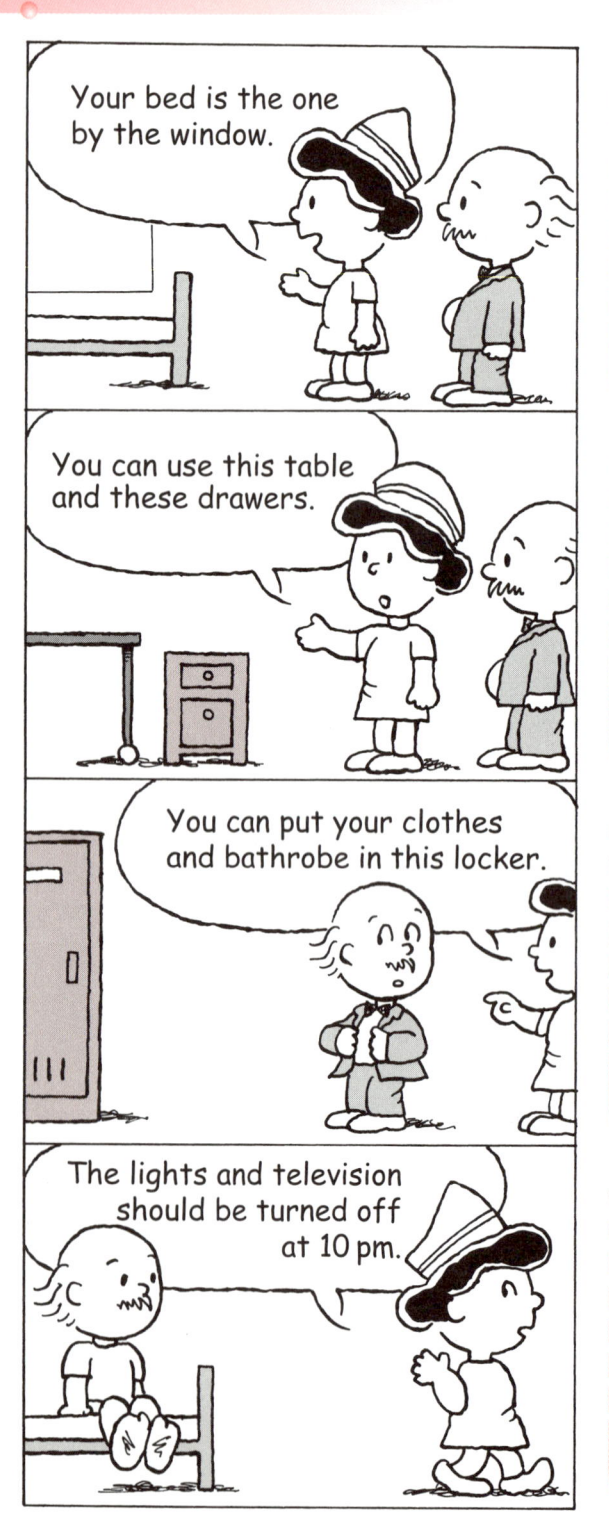

病室にて　　The Patient's Room

Your bed is the one by the window.

N：窓際のベッドをお使いください．

You can use this table and these drawers.

N：このテーブルと引き出しをご使用ください．

You can put your clothes and bathrobe in this locker.

N：洋服やバスローブはこのロッカーの中に入れて下さい．

The lights and television should be turned off at 10 pm.

N：部屋の明かりやテレビは，午後10時に消してください．

📖 Vocabulary をふやそう

bedside table：床頭台

call bell and interphone：呼出ベルとインターフォン

bed control：ベッドコントロール

bed light：ウォールライト

vase：花瓶

television（TV）：テレビ

washbasin：洗面器
ワッシュベイスン

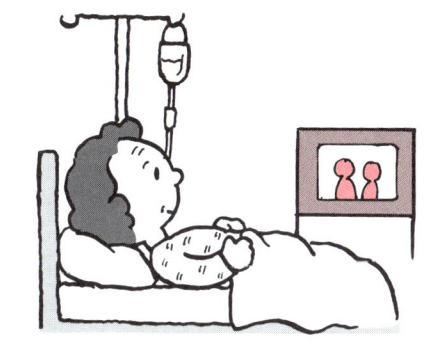

🔳 病棟を案内してみよう！🔳

The toilet is at the end of the hall on the left.
The bath is next to that.

Meal times are 7:30, noon and 5 o'clock.

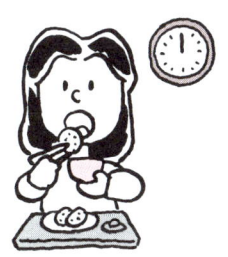

You can't use your cell phone inside the hospital. Please use the public phone, if you need to make a call.

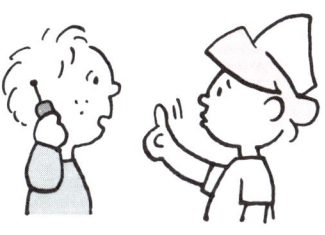

トイレはこの廊下の突き当たりの左側．お風呂はその隣です．

食事時間は7時30分，12時，5時です．

病院の中では携帯電話は使えません．必要の際は公衆電話をお使いください．

Visiting hours are from 3 to 7 pm.
　面会時間は午後3時から7時までです．

You can use the bath between 11 am and 3 pm.
　入浴時間は午前11時から午後3時までです．

Lesson 17-A

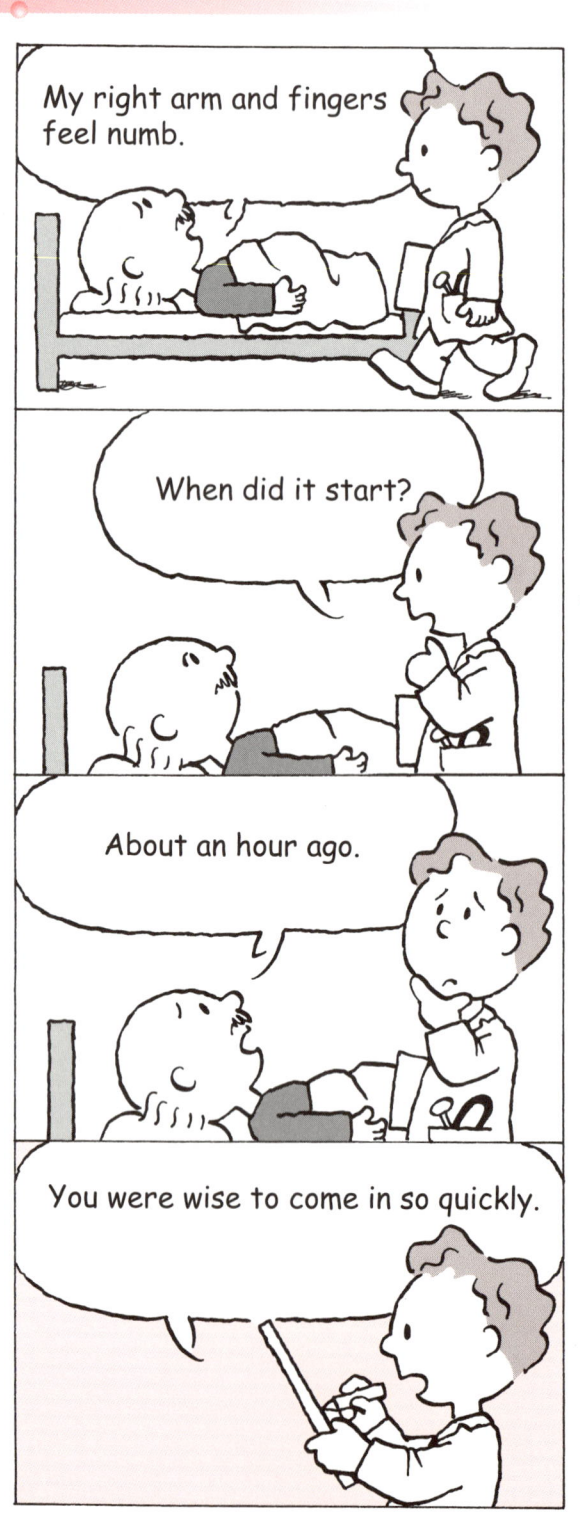

脳卒中 Stroke

My right arm and fingers feel numb.

P：右の腕と指にしびれを感じます．

When did it start?

D：いつから始まりましたか？

👉 When did you notice it?（いつ気づきましたか？）という尋ね方もある．

About an hour ago.

P：ほぼ1時間くらい前からです．

You were wise to come in so quickly.

D：すぐ来ていただいて良かったですよ．

Vocabulary をふやそう

aneurysm：動脈瘤
アンニュリズム

thrombus, clot：血栓，凝血
スランバス　クラットゥ

embolus：栓子
エンボラス

occlusion：閉塞
オクルージョン

abnormal sensation：知覚異常
アブノーマル

paralysis：麻痺
パラリスィス

slurred speech：不明瞭言語
スラードゥ

dysarthria：構音障害
ディスアースリア

aphasia：失語症
アフェージア

anticoagulant：抗凝血薬
アンタイコアーギュラントゥ

physical therapy：物理(理学)療法
セラピー

脳卒中患者の様子

My mouth droops so I can't eat well.
ドゥループス

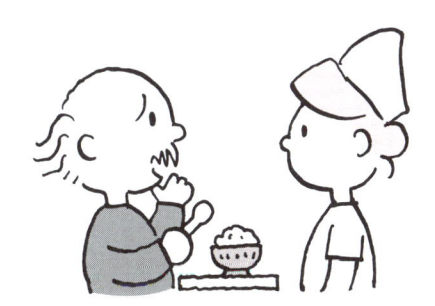

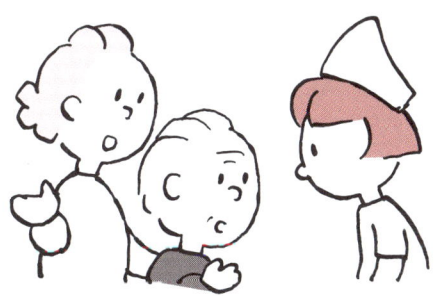

口が垂れてうまく食べられません．

She seems to understand, but she can't reply.

理解しているようなんですが，返事ができません．

She cries from frustration.
フラストゥレイション

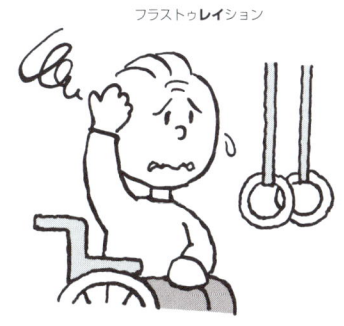

イライラして泣いています．

His leg strength is improving.

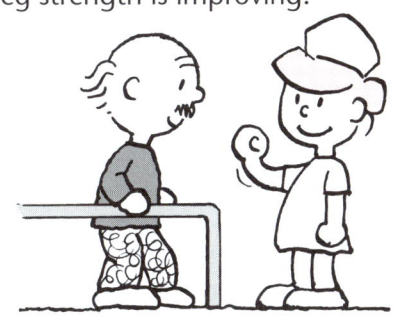

足に力が入るようになってきています．

Lesson 17-B

心臓ペースメーカー / Cardiac Pacemaker

The generator under your collarbone gives off a weak current.

N：鎖骨の下に入れたジェネレーターから弱い電流が流れます．

One wire goes to the upper heart and the other to the lower.

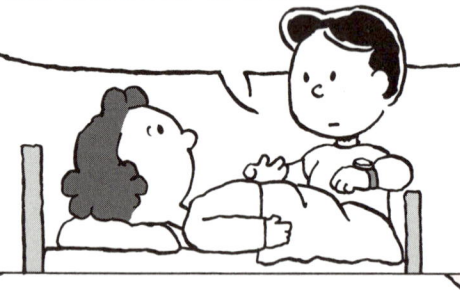

N：ワイヤーの1つは心房へ，もう1つは心室へ行きます．

The current comes on automatically to maintain your heart rate.

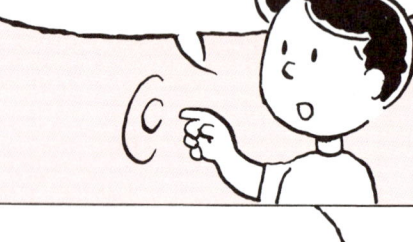

N：電流は心拍数を維持するために自動的に流れるのです．

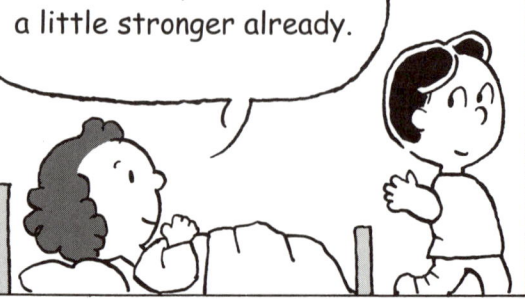

Somehow I feel a little stronger already.

P：なんだか少し体に力が出てきたような気がします．

Vocabulary をふやそう

regurgitation：逆流
リガージィ**テイ**ション

valve：弁
ヴァルヴ

digitalis：ジギタリス
デイジィ**タ**リス

biofeedback：バイオフィードバック(BF)法

atrium：心房
エイトゥリアム

ventricle：心室
ヴェントゥリクル

artery：動脈
アータリー

vein：静脈
ヴェイン

循環器疾患をアセスメントしよう！

Has the doctor told you about a murmur?
　　　　　　　　　　　　　　　　マーマー
医師から心雑音が聞こえると指摘されたことがありますか？

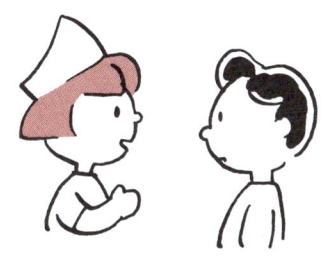

My husband became pale when he climbed stairs at the station.
夫は駅の階段をのぼった際，顔色が真っ青になりました．

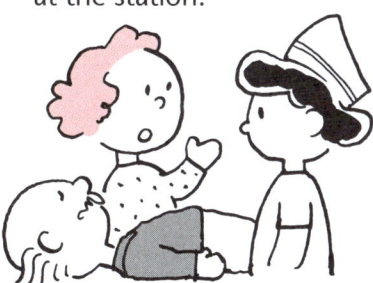

I often feel lightheaded when I work at the office.
　　　　　　ライトゥヘディドゥ
会社で仕事をしているとき，よく頭がふらふらします．

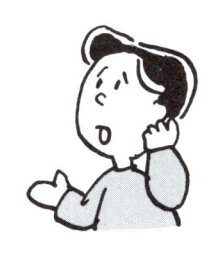

Do you have palpitations?
　　　　　　パルピ**テイ**ションズ
動悸がしますか？

Are you hypertensive or hypotensive?
　　　ハイパー**テン**スィヴ　　ハイポ**テン**スィヴ
高血圧ですか，それとも低血圧ですか？

Do you have chest discomfort?
　　　　　　　　　ディス**カム**フォートゥ
胸部に不快感がありますか？

Do your arms and legs get numb?
　　　　　　　　　　　　　　ナム
手足がしびれますか？

COLUMN　ペースメーカーと携帯電話　Pacemakers and Cell Phones

心臓を収縮させる電気信号を人工的に作り出すペースメーカーは，携帯電話の発する電磁波(electromagnetic waves)によって誤作動し，脈を速めたり遅らせたりする危険性があるため，電車の優先座席付近では通話やメールの送受信が禁じられ，電源を切ることが原則となっています．同様に，医療機器も電磁波の影響を受けるため，病院での使用が禁じられています．なお，電磁波の影響を受けない距離は22cm以上と言われています．

Lesson 18-A

手術の翌朝 / 1st Morning Post-op

> Mr. Russell? I'm sorry to wake you.

N：ラッセルさん，起こしてごめんなさいね．

> I need to suction your throat. Please open your mouth.

N：痰をとりましょう．口を開けてください．

☞ suction は「吸引，吸い出す」という意．痰は phlegm（フレム）あるいは sputum（スピュータム）とも言う．

> My wound hurts.

P：傷口が痛いです．

> I'll get your pain medicine. Later you can try sitting up.

N：痛み止めを打ちましょう．後で起き上がってみましょうね．

☞ 痛み止めは，正式には pain-relief medicine である．

📖 Vocabulary をふやそう

wound, lesion：傷
ウゥンドゥ　リージョン

incision：切開
インスィジョン

stoma, colostomy：ストーマ（人工肛門）
ストウマ　　コラストミー

scar：傷痕
スカー

keloid：ケロイド
キーロイドゥ

skin care：スキンケア

dressing change：包帯や帯具交換
ドゥレッスィング

deep breathing：深呼吸

🎏 術前患者への説明 🎏

We have to shave your surgical area before the operation.

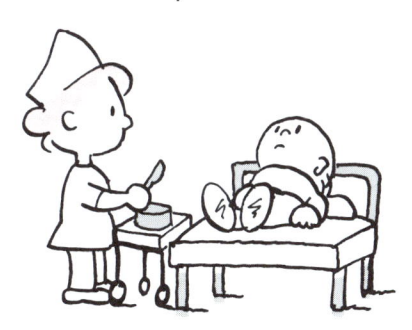

手術の前に手術部位の剃毛をします．

We will start an IV in your arm two hours before surgery.

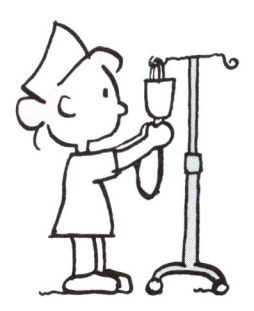

手術の2時間前から点滴を始めます．

We will take you to the operating room on a stretcher.

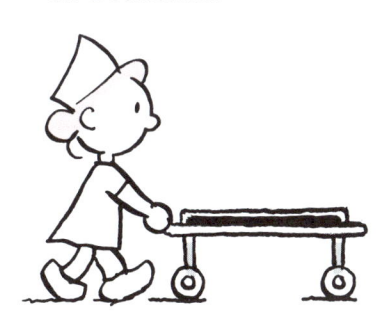

手術室へはストレッチャーで運びます．

We will check your temperature and blood pressure at 7 o'clock in the morning.
　朝7時に体温と血圧を測ります．

You will receive an enema tomorrow morning.
　　　　　　　　　　エネマ
　明日の朝，浣腸をします．

You will go to the recovery room after surgery, and you will go back to your room after you fully wake up.
　術後，回復室に入り，目が充分に覚めたら病室に戻ります．

Lesson 18-B

術後3日 — 3rd Day Post-op

My incision is still really painful.
(インスィジョン)

P：まだ，すごく傷口が痛いです．

Then let's talk with the doctor about increasing your pain medicine.

N：それでは先生に，痛み止めを増やしてもらえるように話してみましょう．

☞ 痛み止めは painkiller ともいう（レッスン6B参照）．

Also, I can't get to sleep.

P：それに眠れないです．

Controlling the pain may help that. If not, we'll see about a sleeping pill.

N：痛みがおさまれば眠れるかもしれません．それでも眠れなかったら，睡眠薬について聞いてみましょう．

📖 Vocabulary をふやそう

esophagus：食道
イソファガス

duodenum：十二指腸
ドゥオディーナム

intestines：腸
インテスティンズ

parenteral nutrition：腸管外栄養
パレンテラル　　ヌートゥリション

intubation：挿管
イントゥベイション

feeding tube：栄養管

liquid diet：流動食

analgesic, painkiller：鎮痛薬
アナルジーズィック

tube feeding：経管栄養

術後患者への対応

This IV contains a painkiller; however, let me know if your pain isn't relieved.

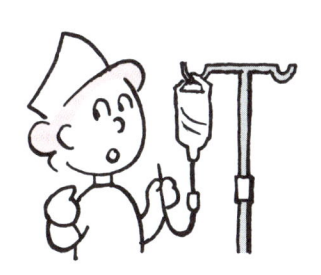

You will be able to sit up tomorrow.
You can walk in three or four days.

You will have a regular diet from tomorrow.

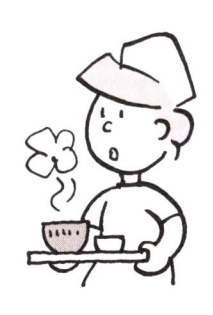

この点滴には痛み止めが入っていますが，痛みが緩和されない場合はおっしゃってください．

明日から起き上がれますよ．
3〜4日したら歩けるでしょう．

明日から普通の食事になります．

COLUMN　アメリカの病院で働く看護師が身につけるもの　What Nurses Wear in America

1990年代初期ごろまで，アメリカでは看護学校を卒業するときに，病院で支給しないナースキャップ(nurse's cap)を学生自らが購入していました．学校や病院が，キャップ着用を要求しない現在では，ほとんどの看護師が被っていません．バッチ(pin)は，今でも看護学校の卒業式にピンズ・セレモニーで支給されています．制服(uniform)の襟や胸に自分の母校のピンをつけるのですが，規則ではないので，付けていない看護師も多いです．白衣もあまり着なくなりました．映画で見る医師が，手術の際に身につける上着とズボンに分かれたものをスクラブ(scrub)と呼び，看護師も着ています．それもデザインが施されていたり，色物です．靴(shoes)も以前のような白い革靴ではなく，ジョギング・シューズを履いている看護師が多くなっています．

Lesson 19-A

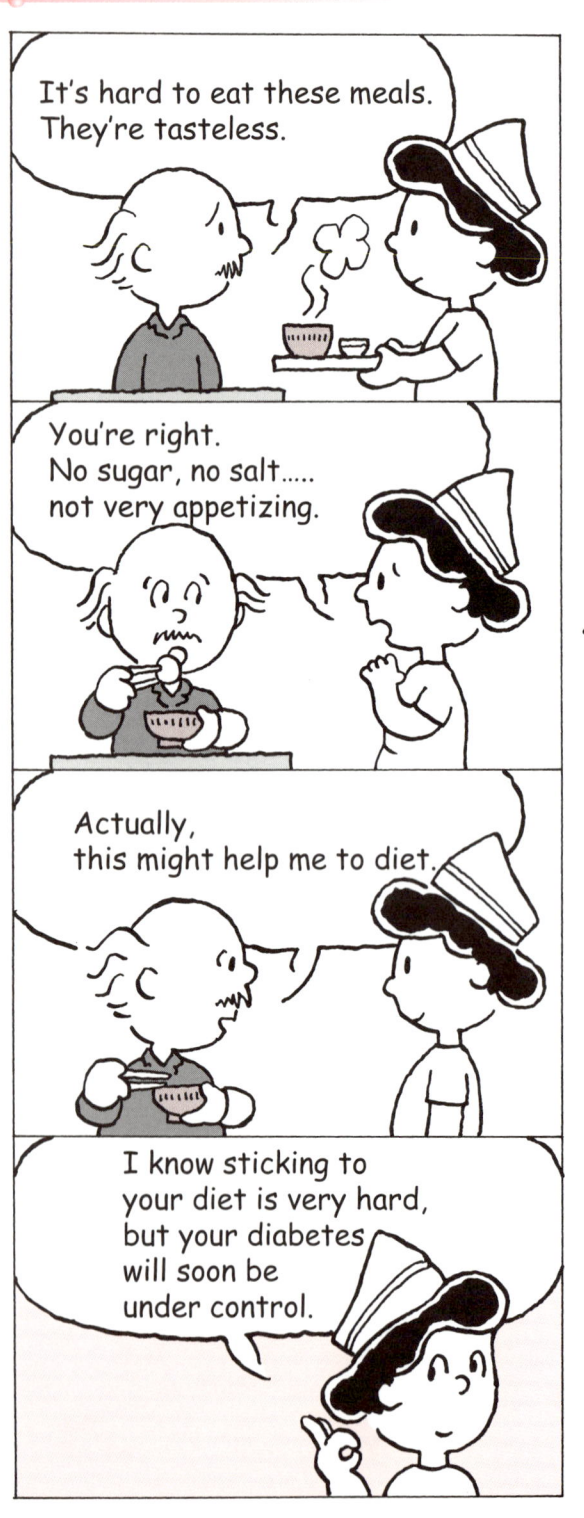

糖尿病 — Diabetes

Panel 1:
It's hard to eat these meals. They're tasteless.

P：ここの食事は食べづらいです．味がなくてねぇ．

Panel 2:
You're right. No sugar, no salt...... not very appetizing.

N：そうですよね．甘みもないし，塩気もないし…あまり，おいしくないですよね．

☞ appetizingは「食欲をそそる，美味な」という意．appetiteは「食欲」のこと．

Panel 3:
Actually, this might help me to diet.

P：実際のところ，これならダイエットになりそうです．

Panel 4:
I know sticking to your diet is very hard, but your diabetes will soon be under control.

N：食事療法はとても大変ですよね，でも，すぐに糖尿病をコントロールできますよ．

📖 Vocabulary をふやそう

overweight, obesity：肥満

lack of exercise：運動不足

stress：ストレス

blood sugar level：血糖値

hypoglycemia：低血糖

diabetic coma：糖尿病性昏睡

insulin shock：インスリン・ショック

injection, shot：注射

urine (blood) test：尿（血液）検査

diabetic retinopathy：糖尿病性網膜症

🔲 糖尿病の症状とアドバイス 🔲

I'm always thirsty.

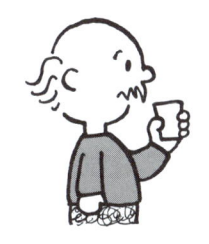

いつも喉が渇きます．

I've gained / lost weight.

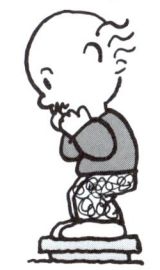

体重が増えました／減りました．

My hands and feet feel numb.

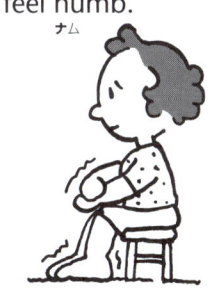

手足がしびれます．

I have palpitations.
My heart flutters.
My heart beats rapidly.

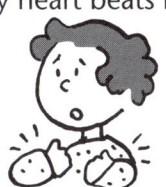

動悸が激しいです．

My vision has decreased.

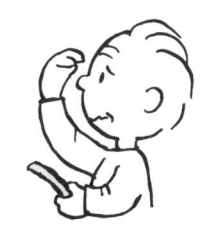

視力が落ちました．

Your weight is 75 kilograms. You should keep your calories down to 2000 per day.
　体重が75キロですので，1日の摂取熱量を2000ぐらいに抑えましょう．

In addition to your medication, more exercise would help.
　薬だけでなく，運動も効果的ですよ．

Reducing animal fat and increasing fiber in your diet is good, too.
　動物性脂肪を減らし，食物繊維をふやすのもいいですよ．

Lesson 19-B

退院指導

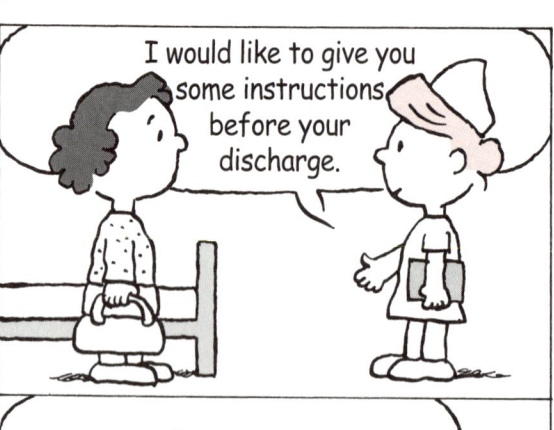

Patient Teaching at Discharge

I would like to give you some instructions before your discharge.

N：退院される前にいくつかお伝えしたいことがあります．

You need to see your doctor once a week for the first month.

N：最初の1か月は週1回受診してください．

☞ 「受診する」は have a check-up，あるいは visit the office ともいう．

This is the prescription. When you leave, please go to the pharmacy in front of this hospital to get the medicine.

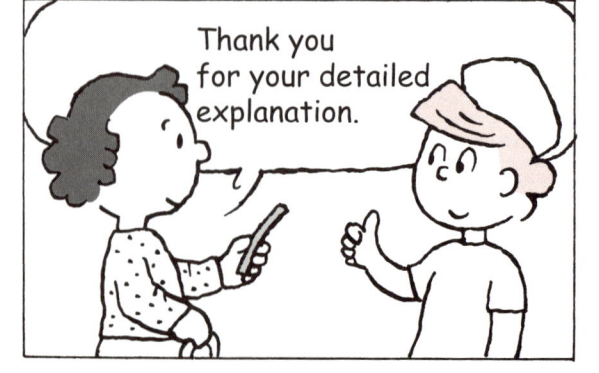

N：これが処方箋です．お帰りになるときに病院の前の薬局で薬を受け取ってください．

Thank you for your detailed explanation.

P：くわしいご説明をありがとうございます．

Vocabulary をふやそう

visiting nurse：訪問看護師

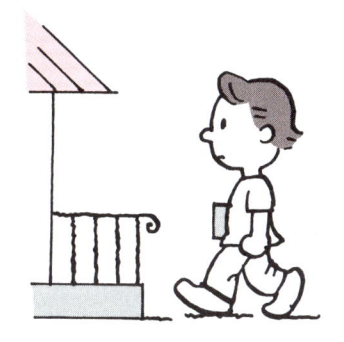

referral letter：紹介状
リファラル

outpatient (counter)：外来（窓口）

insurance premiums：保険料
インシュランス　プリミアムズ

public health nurse：保健師

follow-up：再調査
ファロウアップ

患者教育で使われるフレーズ

Be sure to continue taking your medicine even if you're feeling better.

You have an appointment for next Friday.

Do you want to receive home care?

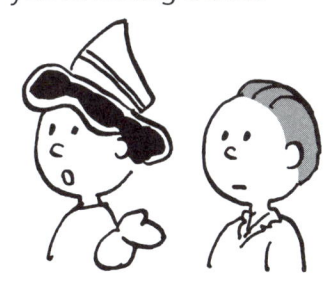

調子が良くなっても薬を飲み続けてくださいね.

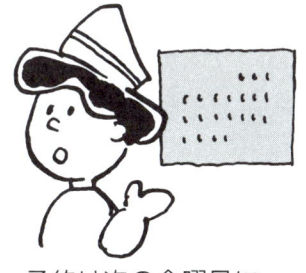

予約は次の金曜日にとれています.

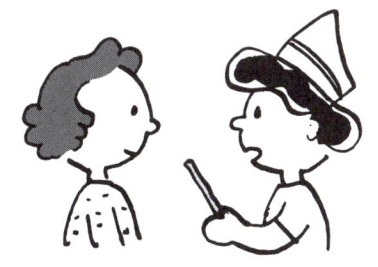

訪問看護をご希望ですか？

You can go back to your work from Friday. Please come to see your doctor regularly.
　　金曜日から職場に復帰できますよ．定期的に受診してくださいね．

COLUMN セラピューティック技術をマスターしよう！ Mastering Therapeutic Technique

糖尿病患者（diabetic patient）が食べ物の味に不平（complain）をこぼしても，すぐに「だめです．食べてください」と言わずに，「そうですよね…」と，患者の思いを一旦受け入れることが大切です（74頁参照）．それから，「でも…」と続けて，回復（recover）するためには，あるいは合併症（complications）を予防（prevent）するためには，そういう食事が必要であるということを伝えます．このようなやり方を英語では，therapeutic（セラピューティック）と言います．看護師は患者との対話の中で，このセラピューティックの技術を用いることで，コミュニケーションをスムーズにできます．

Lesson 20-A

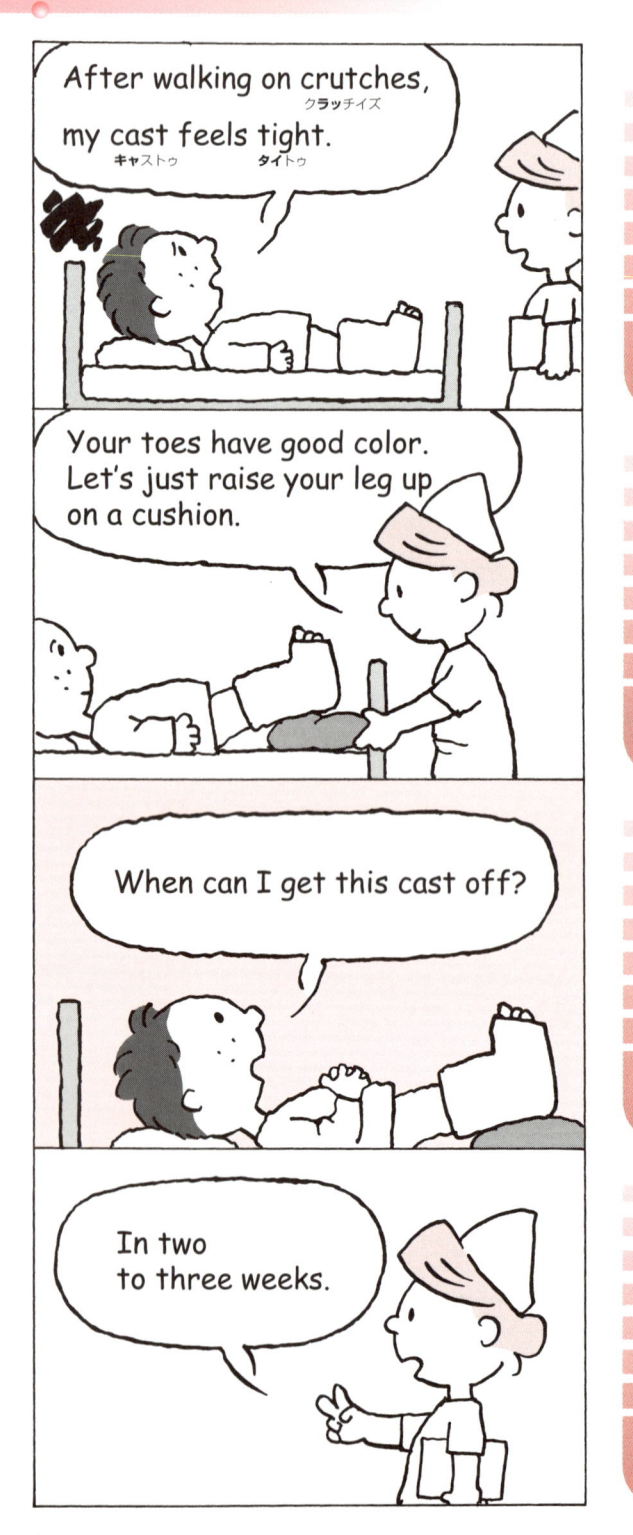

足骨折 — Leg Fracture

After walking on crutches, my cast feels tight.
クラッチイズ キャストゥ タイトゥ

P：松葉杖で歩いたせいか，ギプスがきついです．

Your toes have good color. Let's just raise your leg up on a cushion.

N：足指の色は良いですよ．では，クッションで足を高くしましょう．

When can I get this cast off?

P：いつギプスがとれますか？

In two to three weeks.

N：あと2〜3週間くらいです．

Vocabulary をふやそう

bandage, dressing
バンデェジ

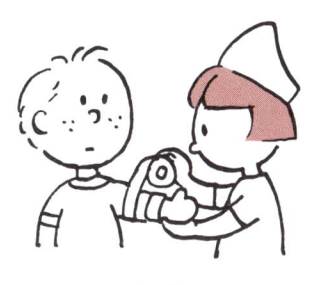

包帯

impaired circulation：循環障害
インペアードゥ　サーキュレイション

pus：膿
パス

traction：牽引
トゥラクション

bedrest：床上安静

orthopedic surgery：整形外科手術
オーソピーディック

リハビリが必要です！

You will need rehabilitation for one or two weeks before your discharge.

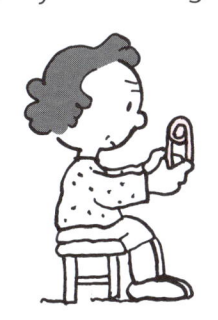

It will be very effective to practice walking every day.

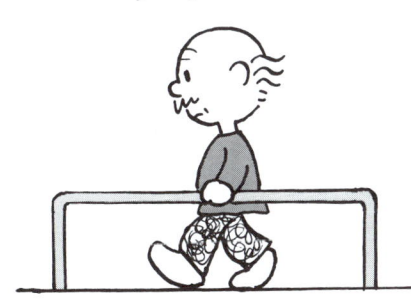

You can use a wheelchair (a pair of crutches) to go to the rehabilitation room.

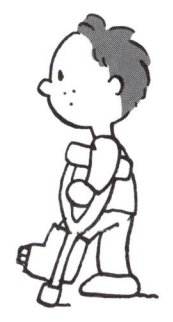

退院する前に1〜2週間のリハビリが必要です．

毎日の歩行訓練はかなり効果がありますよ．

リハビリのお部屋まで車椅子(松葉杖)をお使いください．

You will receive physical therapy after the operation.
　　術後に理学療法を受けることになります．

Just walking to the bathroom is a kind of exercise.
　　洗面所まで歩くだけでも運動になりますよ．

Lesson 20-B

内分泌疾患—バセドウ病　Endocrine Disorder—Graves' Disease

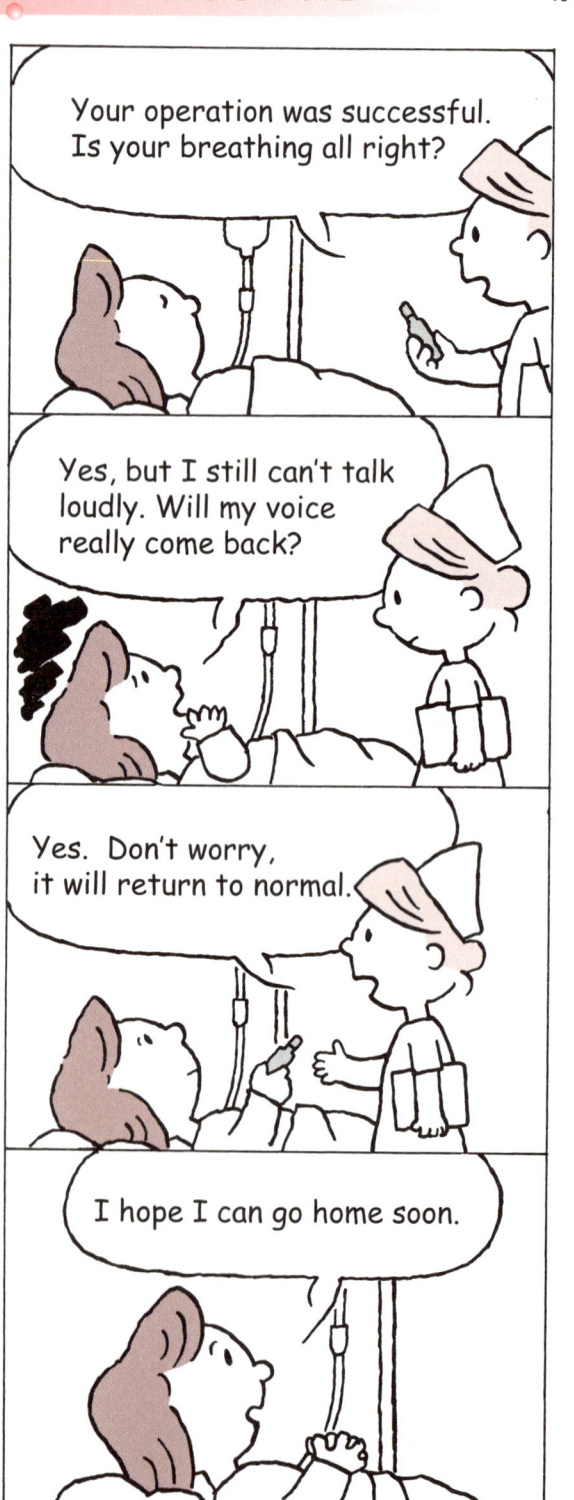

> Your operation was successful. Is your breathing all right?

N：手術は成功でしたよ．呼吸は大丈夫ですか？

> Yes, but I still can't talk loudly. Will my voice really come back?

P：はい，でも，まだ声が出にくいです．ちゃんと元の声に戻るのでしょうか？

> Yes. Don't worry, it will return to normal.

N：大丈夫ですよ．元に戻ると思います．

> I hope I can go home soon.

P：早く退院したいです．

Vocabulary をふやそう

goiter：甲状腺腫
ゴイター

hyperthyroidism：甲状腺機能亢進症
ハイパーサイロイディズム

tachycardia：頻脈
タキカーディア

hoarseness：嗄声（かれ声）
ホースネス　　　させい

radioactive iodine：放射性ヨウ素
レイディオアクティブ　アイオダイン

thyroid crisis：甲状腺中毒症
サイロイド

tracheostomy：気管形成術
トゥレイキアストミー

metabolic rate：代謝率
メタバリック

exophthalmia：眼球突出症
エクソフサルミア

thyroid gland：甲状腺
グランドゥ

内分泌系をアセスメントしよう！

How is your appetite?
Have you gained
or lost weight?

Do you sweat a lot?

My eyes are bulging.
バルジング

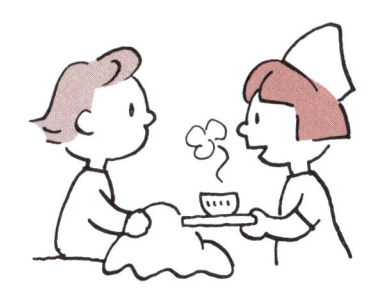

食欲はどうですか？
体重が増えましたか，
それとも減りましたか？

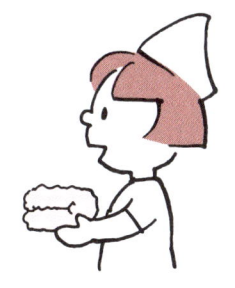

汗をたくさんかきますか？

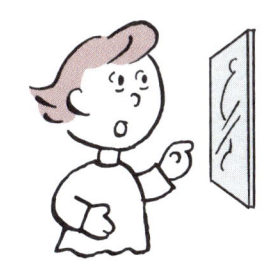

目がふくらんできたわ．

COLUMN 急性肝炎について　Acute Hepatitis

急性肝炎はアルコールや薬などでも発症しますが，主として肝炎ウイルスによる感染症疾患です．現在，ウイルス（virus）は5種類で，日本人の場合，B型，C型が多く，A型肝炎は生の魚介類などから，B型は肝炎ウイルス保持者の血液や性液から，C型は輸血などから感染します．初期症状は黄疸（jaundice）が出て，全身倦怠感（lethargy）と食欲不振（loss of appetite）などです．薬物療法としてはインターフェロンが有効ですが，ウイルスによりインターフェロンが効くものと効かないものがあります．ところで，黄疸は病名ではなくあくまで症状を指す名称です．黄疸が生じるのは，肝臓の機能が低下し，ビリルビン（bilirubin）の代謝が障害されていることを示しています．

Lesson 21-A

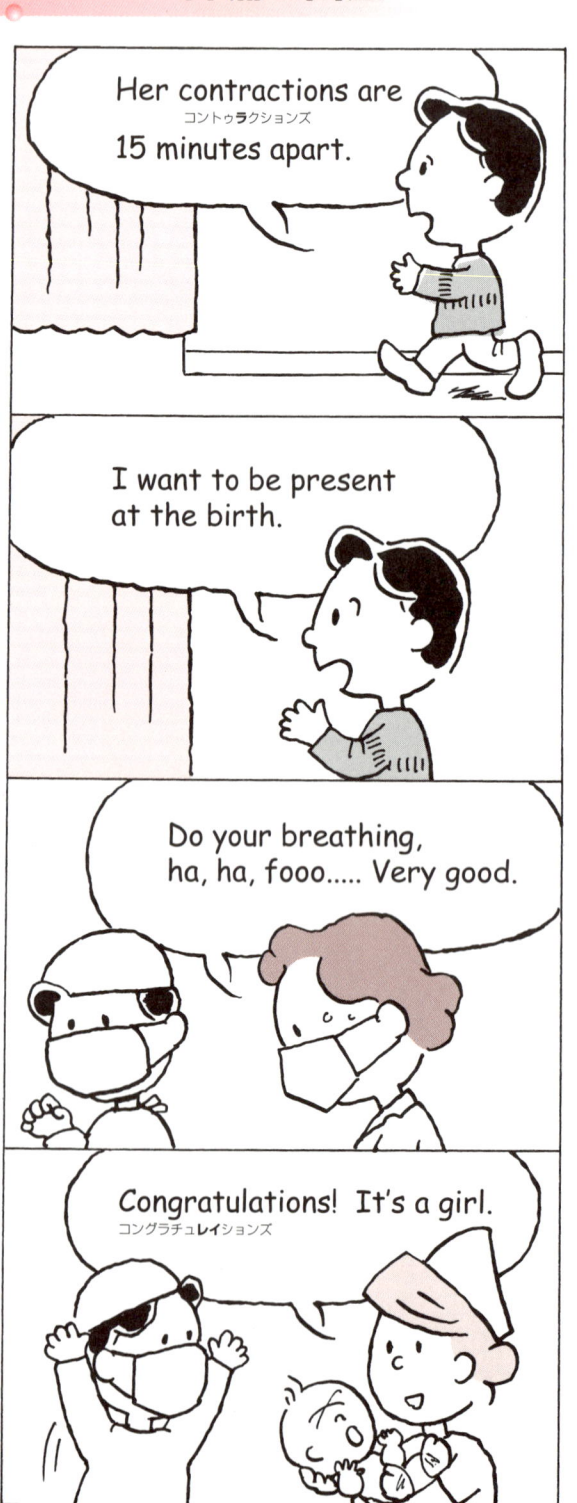

陣痛と出産 — Labor and Delivery

Her contractions are 15 minutes apart.

HB：陣痛が15分間隔です．

I want to be present at the birth.

HB：出産に立ち会わせてください．

Do your breathing, ha, ha, fooo..... Very good.

D：ハッハッフーと息をして…．上手ですよ．

Congratulations! It's a girl.

N：おめでとうございます！女の子ですよ．

📝 Vocabulary をふやそう

midwife：助産師
ミドゥワイフ

obstetrician：産科医
アブステトゥリシャン

delivery room：分娩室
デリヴァリー

episiotomy：会陰切開
エピズィアトミー

cesarean section：帝王切開
スィゼリアン

premature birth：早産
プリマチュアー

low birth weight infant：低出生体重児

induced labor：誘発分娩
インドゥーストゥ

🚩 不安いっぱい新米ママへの対応 🚩

P：My son's weight is lower than at birth.
N：Don't worry, that's only temporary.

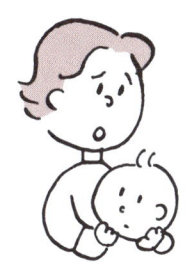

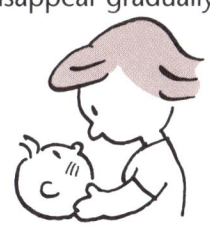

患：出生時より体重が減っています．
看：一時的なものですから，心配ないですよ．

P：My baby doesn't seem to want to breast-feed.
N：Don't be in a hurry.
　　Try to relax, and he'll soon learn how.

患：うまく母乳を飲んでくれません．
看：焦らないで．リラックスしましょう．
　　赤ちゃんは，じきに飲めるようになりますよ．

P：My daughter's face looks a little yellowish.
N：This jaundice happens to most babies
　　ジョーンディス
　　four or five days after they're born.
　　It will disappear gradually.

患：顔が少し黄色いようです．
看：黄疸は生後4〜5日の赤ちゃんに
　　よくみられるものです．
　　そのうち消えますよ．

P：My baby seems to cry more easily than others.
N：Even newborns have their own personality.
　　But if you're worried about it, we can talk with the doctor.

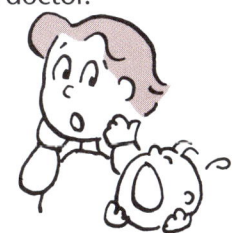

患：よその子よりもよく泣くような気がします．
看：新生児でも，それぞれ性格があるんですよ．
　　ご心配でしたら，医師に相談できますよ．

Lesson 21-B

肝臓の病気 — Liver Disease

This looks very much like cirrhosis.
(スィロスィス)

D：肝硬変の疑いが濃いですね．

But I hardly drink alcohol……
(アルコホール)

P：でも，私はほとんどお酒を飲まないのですが．

☞ hardly は「あまり～しない」という否定の意味を表す単語．

The hepatitis virus is the most likely cause.

D：肝炎ウイルスが原因である確率が高いです．

☞ the most likely cause で「最も可能性の高い原因」という意．

You need to do admission procedures. Would you please come with me?

N：入院の手続きをしなければなりません．こちらへ来ていただけますか？

Vocabulary をふやそう

type A（B, C）hepatitis：A(B,C)型肝炎
ヘパ**タイ**ティス

carrier：保菌者
キャリアー

jaundice：黄疸
ジョーンディス

fatigue：疲労
ファ**ティー**グ

vaccine：ワクチン
ヴァク**スィー**ン

immune serum globulin（ISG）：免疫血清グロブリン
イ**ミュー**ン　　**ス**ィラム　　グ**ラ**ビュリン

isolation：隔離
アイソ**レイ**ション

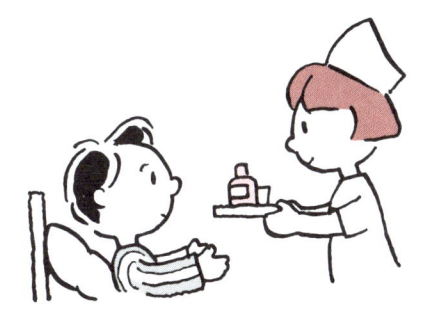

肝臓に問題のある患者をアセスメントしよう 1

About how many drinks do you have a day?

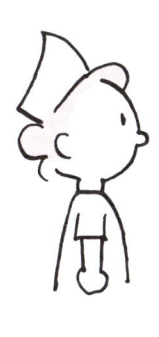

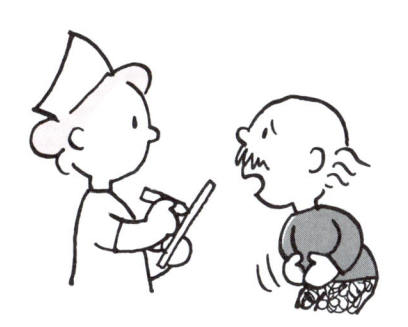

1日にどのくらいアルコールを飲みますか？

Did your pain begin gradually or suddenly?

痛みは徐々に始まりましたか, それとも突然でしたか？

Does the pain go through to your back?
　痛みは背中まで広がりますか

When does the pain happen, before meals or after meals?
　いつ痛みますか？ 食前ですか, それとも食後ですか？

85

Lesson 22-A

肺炎 — Pneumonia

Mr. Takahashi, is my grandpa okay?

He's much better. The antibiotics have brought his fever down.
アンタイバイアティックス

Thank you. I'm so glad.

But he's elderly, and we'll have to be watchful.

FM：高橋さん，うちのおじいちゃんは大丈夫でしょうか？

N：ずいぶんよくなりましたよ．抗生物質で熱が下がったので大丈夫でしょう．

FM：ありがとうございます．よかったわ．

N：ただご高齢でもありますので，私たちは注意しています．

📖 Vocabulary をふやそう

cough：咳
コフ

bloody sputum：血痰
スピュータム

hemoptysis：喀血
ヒマプティスィス

pulmonary edema：肺水腫
プルモナリー　エディマ

pleurisy：胸膜炎
プルリスィー

pneumococcus：肺炎球菌
ヌーモカカス

aspiration：呼吸（息を吸い込むこと），吸引，誤嚥
アスピレイション

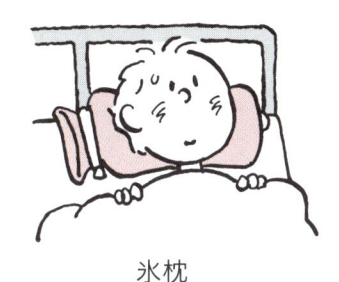

ice pillow

氷枕

🏥 呼吸器疾患患者への対応

I often wheeze, and
ウィーズ
sometimes I have a pain in my chest.

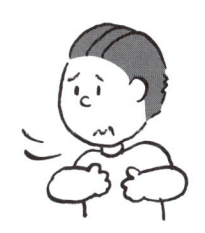

よく息がぜいぜいして，
ときどき胸痛が起こります．

Do you have a cough?
コフ

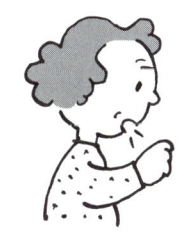

咳をしますか？

Do you have shortness of breath?
ブレス
Have you ever had asthma?
アズマ

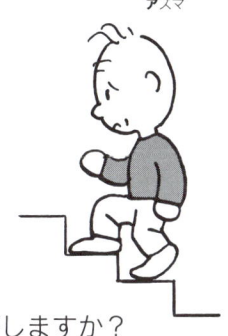

息切れがしますか？
喘息になったことがありますか？

Has your son ever had pneumonia or bronchitis?
　　　　　　　　　　　　ヌモウニア　　　ブロンカイティス
　息子さんは肺炎や気管支炎にかかったことがありますか？

I coughed up blood.
　痰に血が混じっていました．

87

Lesson 22-B

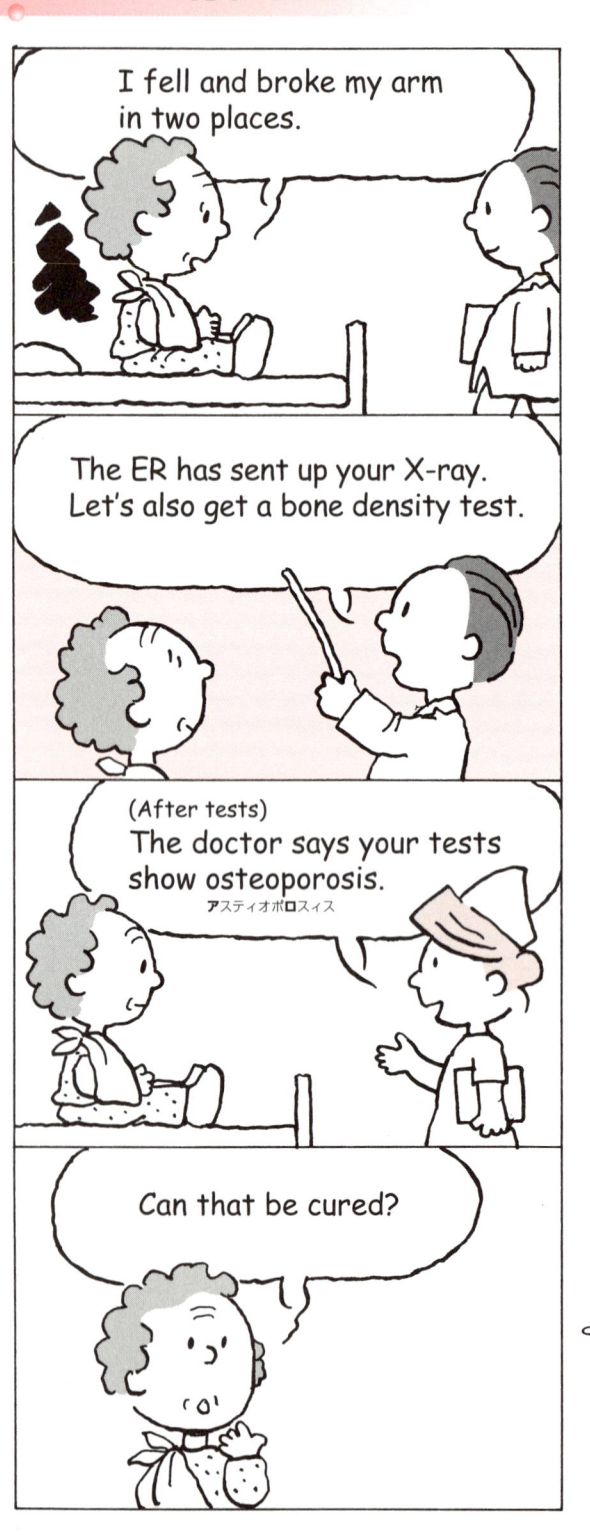

骨粗鬆症　Osteoporosis

I fell and broke my arm in two places.

P：転んだら腕を2箇所骨折しました．

The ER has sent up your X-ray. Let's also get a bone density test.

D：救急室からレントゲン写真をもらいました．骨密度も測定してみましょう．

(After tests) The doctor says your tests show osteoporosis.
アスティオポロスィス

（検査後）
N：検査の結果，先生は骨粗鬆症と言っていますよ．

Can that be cured?

P：それは治るのでしょうか？

☞ 「治る」には色々な言い方がある．heal, recover from, get over など．

📖 Vocabulary をふやそう

aging：加齢

spinal fractures：脊椎骨折
スパイナル フラクチュアーズ

spontaneous fractures：特発性骨折
スパンテイニアス

hormone replacement therapy (HRT)
ホーモウン　　　　　　　　セラピー
　　　　　　　　　：ホルモン療法

weight-bearing exercise：加重負荷運動
ベアリング

calcium：カルシウム
キャルスィアム

dairy products：乳製品
デェリー

bisphosphonates：ビスフォスフォネート製剤
ビスファスフォネイツ

🎌 日常生活についてアセスメントしてみよう！🎌

What time do you usually go to bed (wake up)?

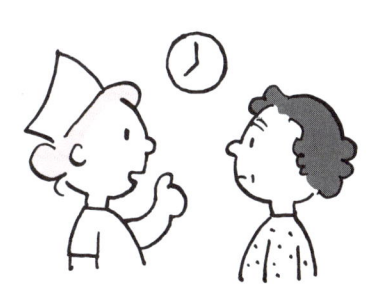

いつも何時に就寝（起床）しますか？

Do you have difficulty getting to sleep?

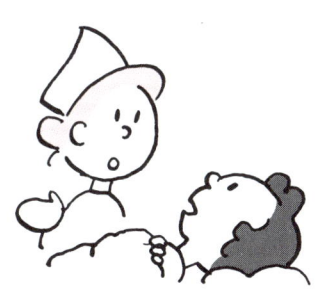

寝付きにくいですか？

How often do you have a bowel movement?

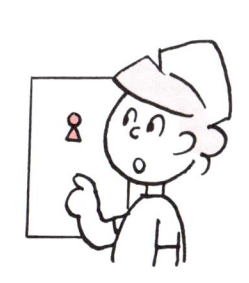

どのくらいの頻度で便通がありますか？

Do you live alone or with your family?
　一人住まいですか，それともご家族とお住まいですか？

Do you have anyone who takes care of you?
　あなたの世話をしてくれる人がいますか？

Is there any problem with your appetite?
　食欲に何か問題はありますか？

How often do you go out to eat per week?
　週に何回くらい外食しますか？

Do you get constipation or diarrhea easily?
　　　　　　カンスティペイション　　　ダイアリア
　便秘しやすいですか，それとも下痢しやすいですか？

Lesson 23-A

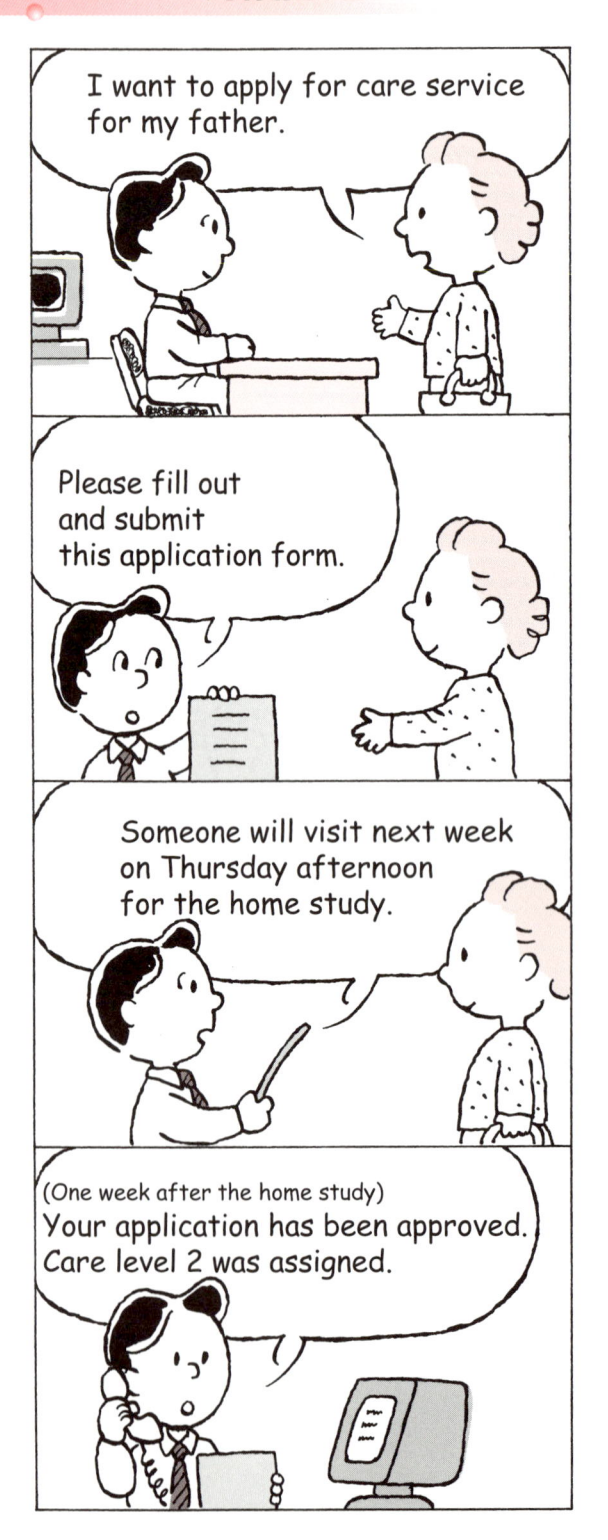

介護認定 — Care Designation

FM: 父の介護サービスの申請をしたいのですが．

CE: この申請書に記入して提出してください．

CE: 来週の木曜の午後，訪問調査をさせていただきます．

（訪問調査から1週間後）
CE: 認定の結果，要介護2と認定されました．

Vocabulary をふやそう

elderly person, senior citizen：高齢者
　　　　　　　　　スィニアー

caregiver：介護者

care recipient：要介護者
　　リスィピエント

care manager：ケアマネジャー

assessment：アセスメント，審査，判定

home renovation：住宅改修
　　レノヴェイション

long-term care insurance：介護保険
　　　　　インスュランス

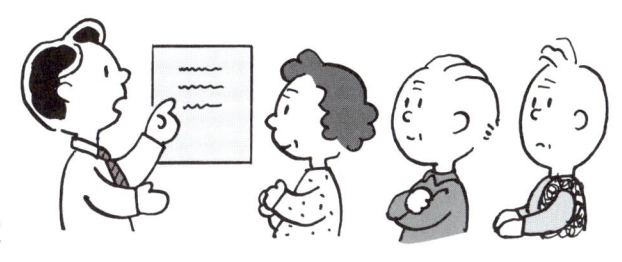

介護保険制度とは？

The present long-term care insurance system began in 2000.
　現在の介護保険制度は平成12年にスタートしました．

When someone becomes 40 years old, he or she must sign up for long-term care insurance.
　40歳になると介護保険に加入しなければなりません．

If anyone in the family needs care, it is provided at only 10% of the cost.
　家族の誰かがサービスを利用したら，費用の1割のみの負担になります．

The types of equipment you can rent using long-term care insurance are determined by law.
　介護保険でレンタルできる用品の基準は法律で定められています．

COLUMN デイサービスとデイケアの違い　"Day Service" vs. "Day Care"

デイサービスは，体の弱い高齢者や軽い痴呆（dementia）の高齢者が部屋に閉じこもらないよう，軽い体操やゲーム，お風呂や食事を一緒にして，人とふれあいながら心を活性するための場です．一方デイケアは，脳血管障害（cerebrovascular disorder；CVD）や骨折（fracture），痴呆の高齢者がリハビリをする場です．理学療法士（physical therapist；PT）や作業療法士（occupational therapist；OT）によって歩行訓練やロープの牽引などが行われますが，折り紙やぬり絵，ボールゲームなどもリハビリの一環として取り入れられることがあります．

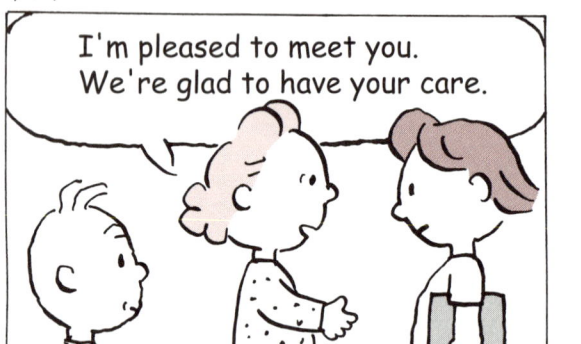

Lesson 23-B

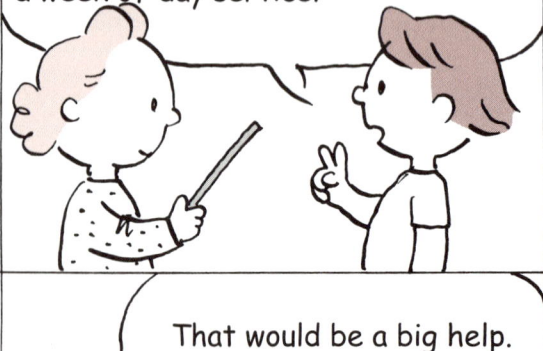

在宅ケア—認知症 / Home Care—Dementia

FM: 初めまして．お世話になります．
I'm pleased to meet you. We're glad to have your care.

CM: 田中さんは介護度2で軽い認知症(ディメンシャ)がありますね．
Mr. Tanaka is assigned care level 2 and has mild dementia, is that right?

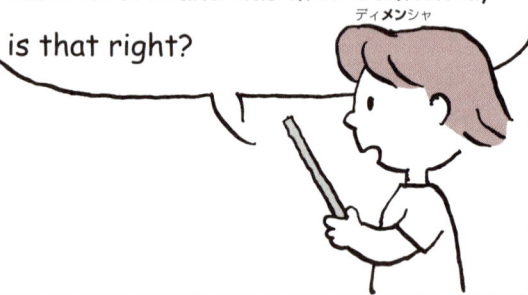

CM: ご家族の負担も考えて，まず週2日のデイサービスはいかがですか？
Considering the burden on the family, how about starting with two days a week of day service?

FM: それは大変助かります．
That would be a big help.

Vocabulary をふやそう

home care：在宅ケア

house call：往診

oxygen concentrator：酸素濃縮器

nasal cannula：経鼻カニューレ
ネイザル　キャンニュラ

oxygen mask：酸素マスク

insomnia, sleeplessness：不眠（症）
インサムニア

turning：寝返り

pressure sore, decubitus ulcer：褥瘡，床ずれ
　　　　　　　　ディキュビタス　　アルサー

terminal care：ターミナルケア

薬の使い方を指示してみよう

Take these tablets / pills / capsules after every meal.

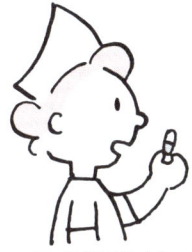

毎食後，この錠剤／カプセルを飲んでください．

Apply this ointment where it itches.
オイントゥメントゥ

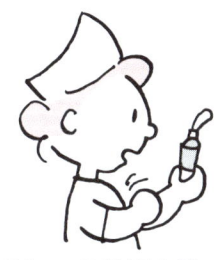

かゆいところにこの軟膏を塗ってください．

Spray once in each nostril
ナストゥリル
morning and evening.

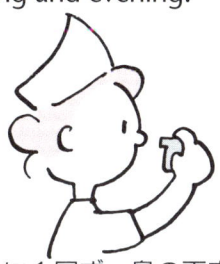

朝と晩に１回ずつ鼻の両穴にスプレーしてください．

Put one or two drops in each eye per day.

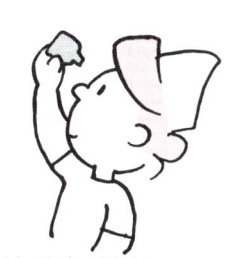

１日１回，それぞれの眼に１～２滴点眼してください．

Take this liquid medicine / powder before meals.
　食前にこの水薬／粉薬を飲んでください．

Place this heat pack where it hurts.
　痛むところにこの温湿布を貼ってください．

This is a rectal suppository. Do not take it orally.
レクタル　　サパズィトリー
　これは坐薬なので，口に入れないでください．

Lesson 24-A

訪問介護―入浴サービス　Home Care—Bath Service

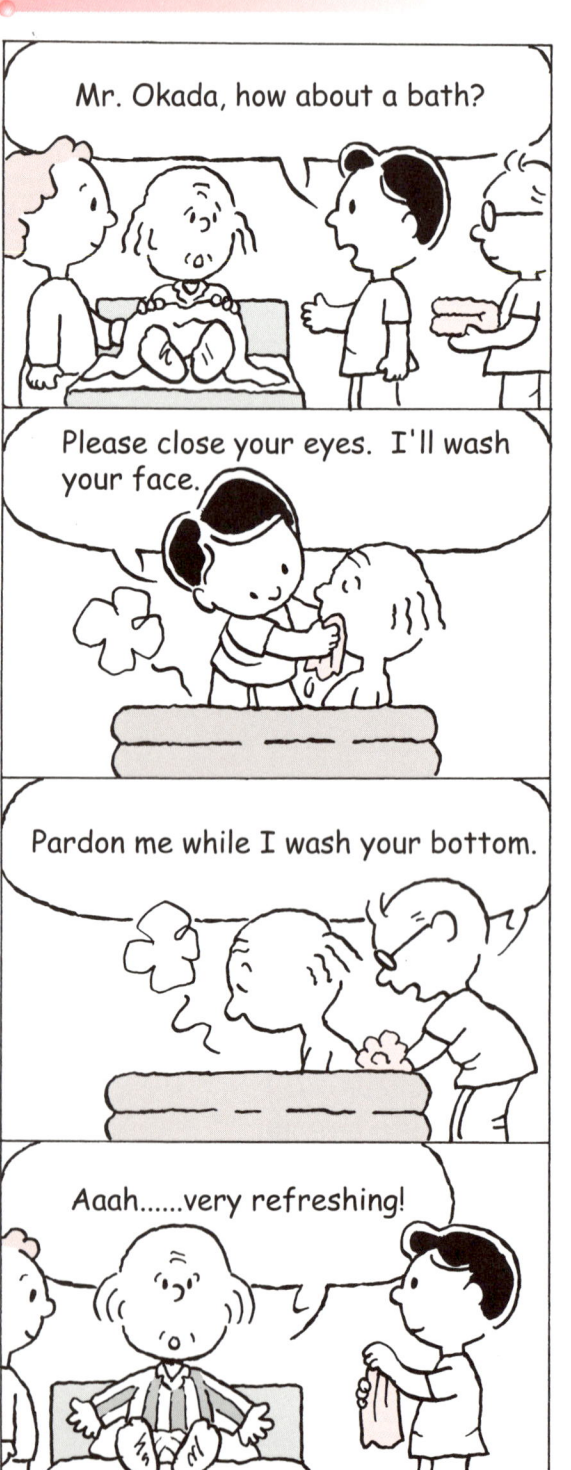

Mr. Okada, how about a bath?

HH1：岡田さん，お風呂に入りましょうか？

Please close your eyes. I'll wash your face.

HH1：目をつぶってください．顔を洗います．

Pardon me while I wash your bottom.

HH2：失礼します．おしりを洗いますね．

Aaah……very refreshing!

P：あ～さっぱりした！

Vocabulary をふやそう

home helper：ホームヘルパー

restlessness：情動不安

agitation：興奮
アジ**テイ**ション

wandering：徘徊

incontinence：失禁
イン**カン**ティネンス

protective pants：おむつ

absorbent pad：尿とりパッド
アブ**ソー**ベントゥ

portable toilet, commode：ポータブルトイレ
コ**モウ**ドゥ

waterproof sheet：防水シート

日常介助のフレーズ

I'm going to give you a bedbath.
ベッドゥバス

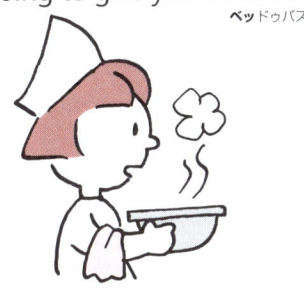

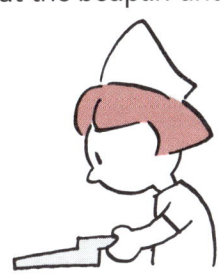

体を拭きましょう．

Please rinse your mouth.

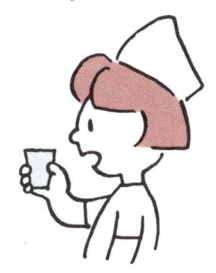

口の中をゆすいでください．

Please lift your bottom.
I will put the bedpan under it.

腰を浮かしてください．
便器を入れます．

Here is your tray.
Would you like to start with soup or salad?

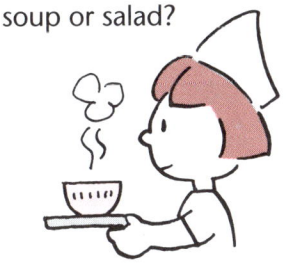

お食事ですよ．
スープから食べ始めますか，
それともサラダですか？

First, I will wash your face with a hot towel, and then your arms.
　最初に熱いタオルで顔を拭き，それから腕を拭きましょう．

Is the water warm enough?
　湯加減はいかがですか？

Please chew well. Are you full? I'll take away your tray.
　よくかんでくださいね．もうおなかいっぱいですか？トレーをお下げしますね．

Lesson 24-B

デイサービス / Day Service

Everybody come together and form a circle.

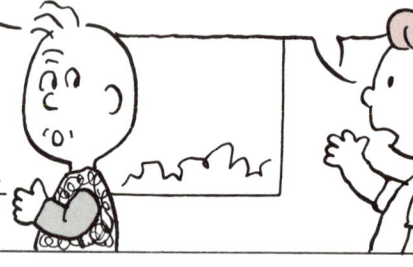

H：皆さんこちらに来て，輪を作ってください．

Please sit down. Today let's play a new game.

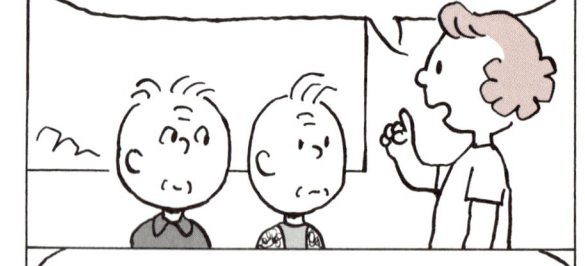

H：どうぞ座ってください．今日は新しいゲームをしましょう．

Hold the big balloon over your head and pass it quickly to the person on your left.

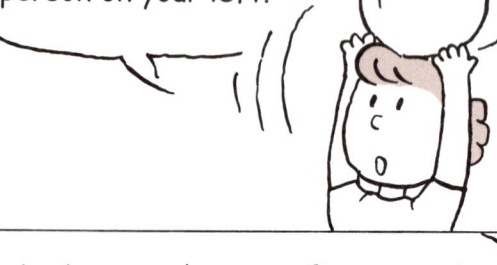

H：頭の上で右回りに，この風船を速く回しましょう．

☞ 時計回りという表現は，clockwise という言葉がある．

A minute and twenty-five seconds. Can you beat that?

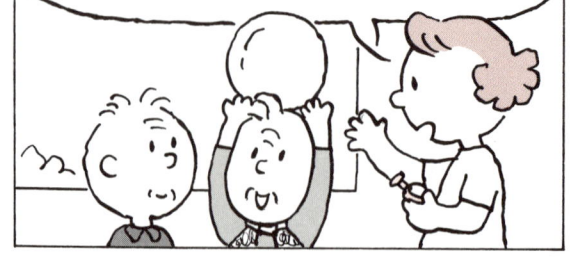

H：1分25秒かかりましたよ．この記録を破れるかしら？

📖 Vocabulary をふやそう

van, shuttle bus：バン，シャトルバス
ヴァン　シャトゥル　バス

dayroom：デイルーム

cane：ステッキ
ケイン

walker：歩行器

(electric) wheelchair：(電動)車椅子

barrier-free：バリアフリー

independence, self-reliance：自立
　　　　　　　セルフ　リライアンス

🌸 いろんな活動で話しかけてみよう 🌸

● Gardening

Do you know the name of this plant?
　この植物の名前をご存知ですか？

What types of flowers do you like?
　どんなお花がお好きですか？

How do you grow this plant?
　この植物をどのように育てるのですか？

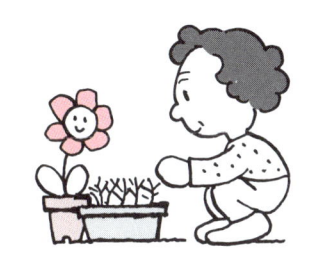

● Arts and Crafts

What can we make with these materials?
　これらの材料でどうするのですか？

That looks like fun. May I join you?
　楽しそうですね．参加しても良いですか？

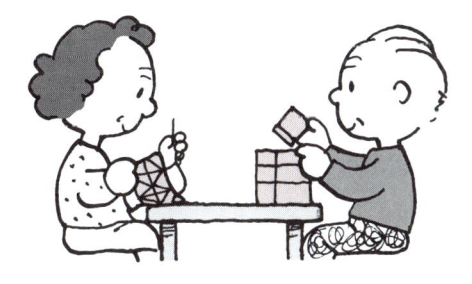

● Croquet / Gateball

Whose turn? Ah! Mr. Tanaka! Good luck.
　誰の番ですか？　あ〜田中さんね．がんばって．

What was your best score?
Who is the best player?
　最高のスコアについて教えてください．
　最高のプレイヤーは誰ですか？

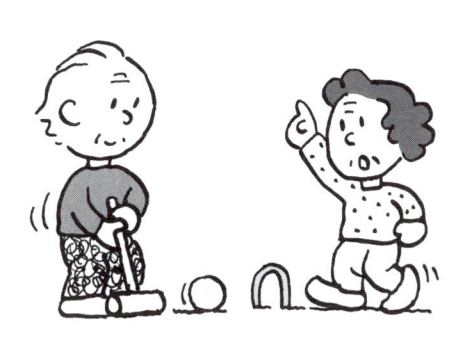

97

Lesson 25-A

介護老人保健施設(老健) Health Maintenance Nursing Home

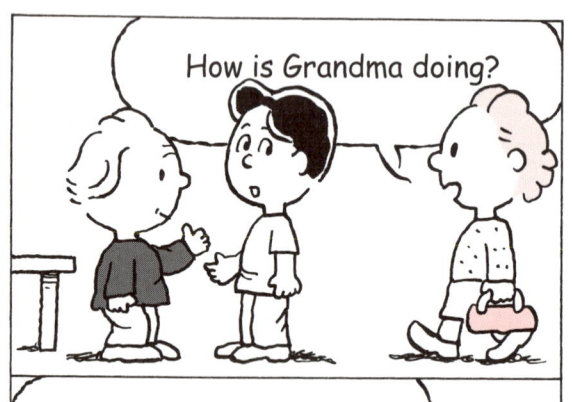

How is Grandma doing?

FM：うちのおばあちゃん，どうでしょうか？

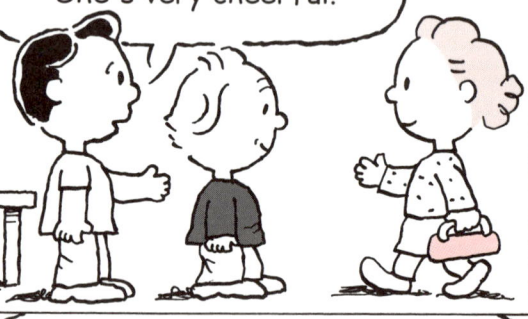

She's very cheerful.

H：とてもお元気ですよ．

This morning she ate all of her breakfast.

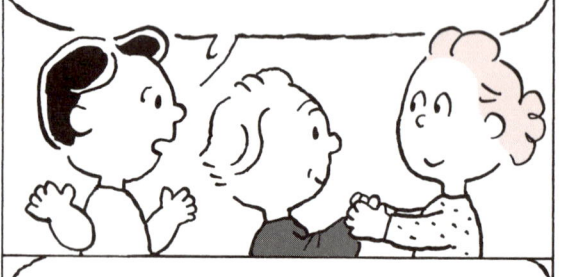

H：今朝，朝食を全部召し上がりましたよ．

Does she say she wants to go home?

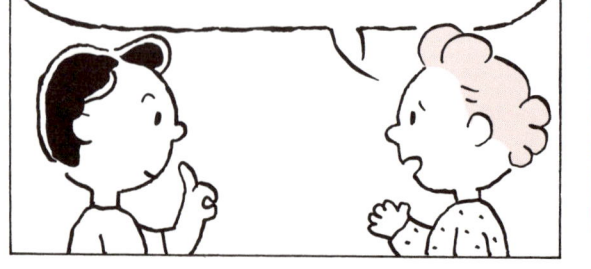

FM：家へ帰りたいと言いませんか？

📖 Vocabulary をふやそう

hard of hearing, partially deaf：難聴

hearing aid：補聴器

complication：合併症
カンプリケイション

rehabilitation：リハビリ

counseling：カウンセリング

balanced diet：バランスの取れた食事

vitamins：ビタミン
ヴァイタミンズ

seeing eye dog, guide dog：盲導犬

よくある高齢者の訴え

Lately I'm forgetful.

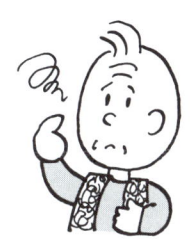

最近，よく物忘れをします．

I can't see clearly.
/ I have bleary eyes.
ブリアリー

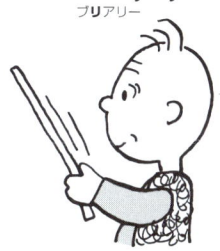

よく物が見えません．
/ 目がかすみます．

I need to urinate very often.
ユリネイトゥ

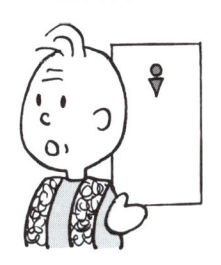

トイレが近いです．

I have difficulty hearing.

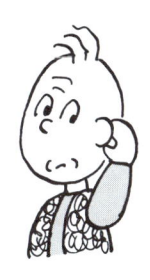

耳が聞こえにくいです．

My balance isn't good.
  バランスが良くないのです．

I'm afraid of falling.
  転びそうで心配です．

Lesson 25-B

介護老人福祉施設（特養）　Long-Term Care Nursing Home

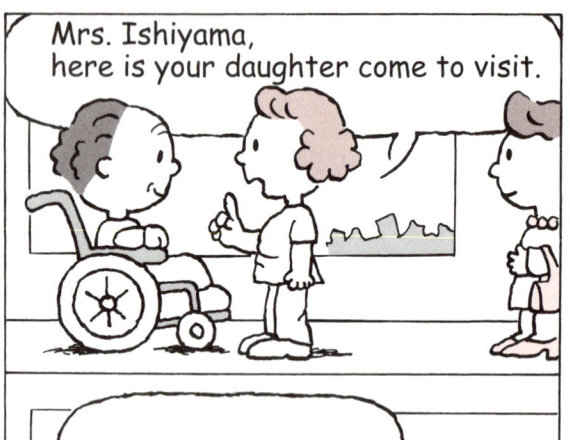

Mrs. Ishiyama, here is your daughter come to visit.

N：石山さん，娘さんが会いにいらっしゃったわよ．

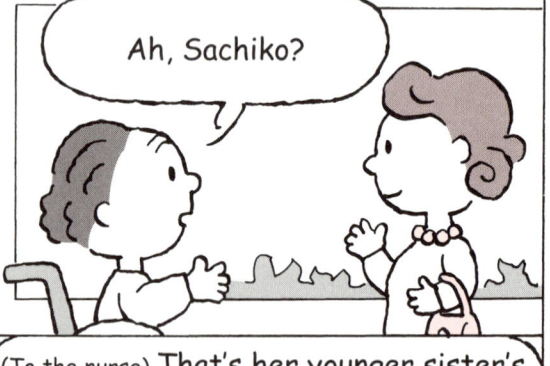

Ah, Sachiko?

P：あぁ，幸子なの？

(To the nurse) That's her younger sister's name. (To her mother) I'm Ayako. How are you feeling?

FM：（看護師に向かって）おばあちゃんの妹の名前です．（母親に向かって）彩子よ．元気にしている？

Pretty good. Are we going for a walk?

Sure, let's go!

P：元気だよ．散歩に行くかい？
FM：いいわよ，行きましょう．

Vocabulary をふやそう

undernourishment, malnutrition：低栄養
アンダーナーリッシュメントゥ　　マルヌートゥリション

hygiene：衛生
ハイジーン

sanitation：衛生施設
サニテイション

stroke：脳卒中，脳溢血
ストゥロウク

bedridden：寝たきり
ベッドゥリドゥン

restraints：抑制，拘束
リストゥレインツ

bedrail：ベッド柵
ベッドゥレイル

level of consciousness：意識レベル
　　　　　カンシャスネス

褥瘡予防

Elderly persons tend to develop bedsores easily, so we have to change their position frequently.

　高齢者は褥瘡ができやすいので，
　頻繁に体位変換をする必要があります．

　💡 褥瘡（床ずれ）はpressure soreともいう．(Lesson23-B 参照)．日本の臨床ではデクビ（decubitusの略）が使われる．

Elderly persons may have loss of appetite. Poor nutrition and weight loss help bedsores develop.

　高齢者は食欲不振になることがあります．
　栄養不足と体重減少から褥瘡ができやすいのです．

When we find a red spot, we rub ointment there.
We may also use an alternating-pressure mattress or cushion.

　赤いところを見つけたら，そこに軟膏を塗ります．
　エアマットやクッションを使うこともあります．

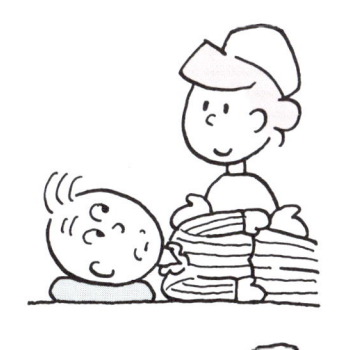

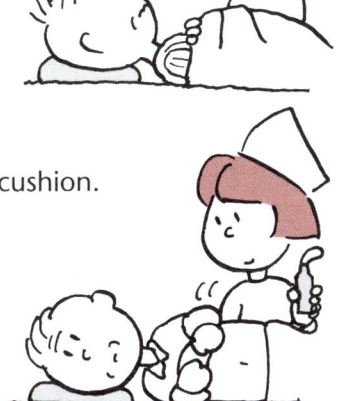

資料　高齢者支援ネットワーク　Senior Citizen's Support Network

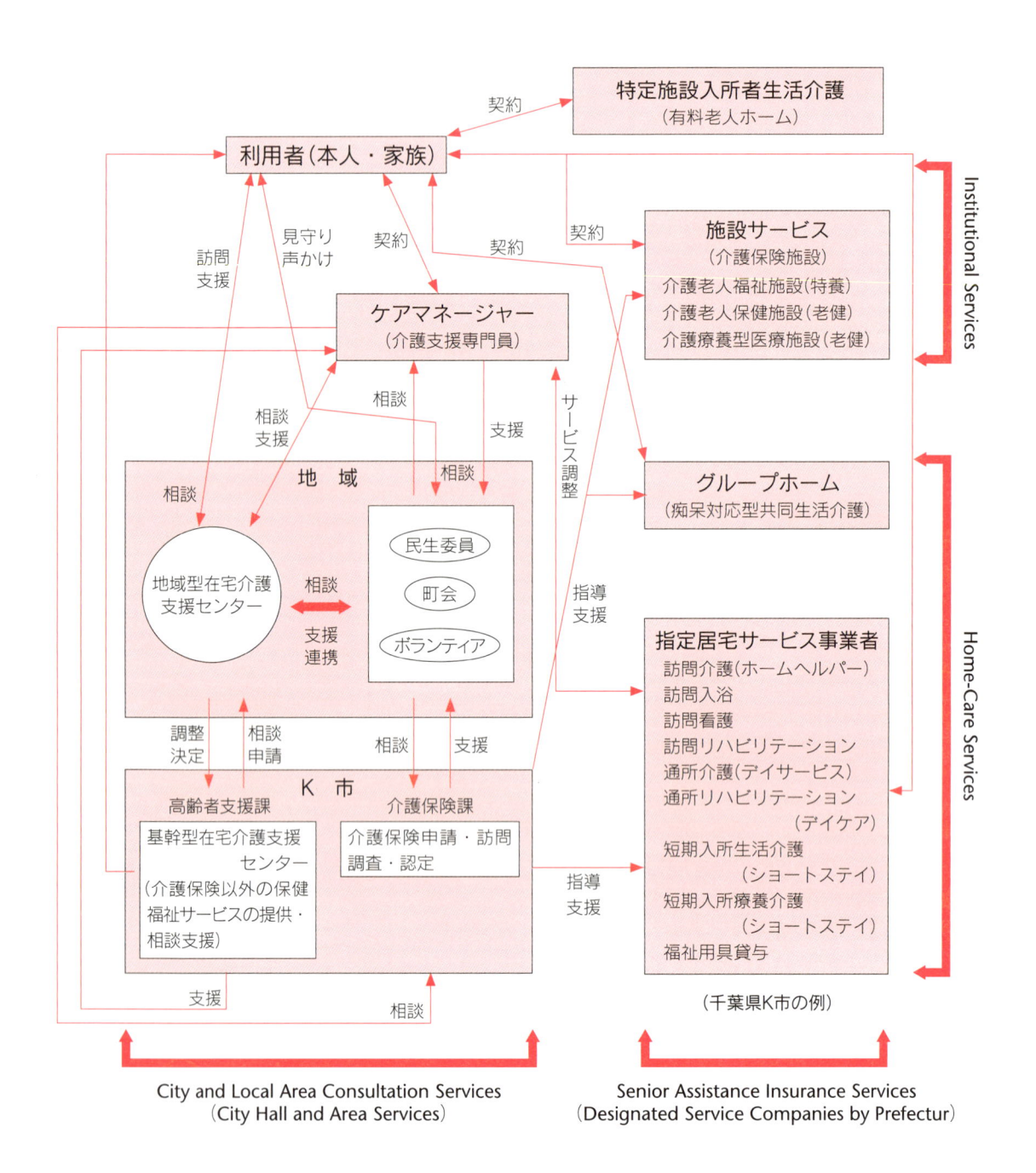

Institutional Services

- 特定施設入所者生活介護（有料老人ホーム）
- 施設サービス（介護保険施設）
  - 介護老人福祉施設（特養）
  - 介護老人保健施設（老健）
  - 介護療養型医療施設（老健）
- グループホーム（痴呆対応型共同生活介護）

Home-Care Services

- 指定居宅サービス事業者
  - 訪問介護（ホームヘルパー）
  - 訪問入浴
  - 訪問看護
  - 訪問リハビリテーション
  - 通所介護（デイサービス）
  - 通所リハビリテーション（デイケア）
  - 短期入所生活介護（ショートステイ）
  - 短期入所療養介護（ショートステイ）
  - 福祉用具貸与

（千葉県K市の例）

利用者（本人・家族） — 契約

ケアマネージャー（介護支援専門員）

地域
- 地域型在宅介護支援センター
- 民生委員
- 町会
- ボランティア

K市
- 高齢者支援課
  - 基幹型在宅介護支援センター（介護保険以外の保健福祉サービスの提供・相談支援）
- 介護保険課
  - 介護保険申請・訪問調査・認定

関係語：訪問支援／見守り声かけ／契約／相談／支援／相談支援／サービス調整／指導支援／調整決定／相談申請／支援連携

City and Local Area Consultation Services
(City Hall and Area Services)

Senior Assistance Insurance Services
(Designated Service Companies by Prefectur)

- 病院を退院する高齢者に対し，上図中のサービスが市役所を中心に用意されている．
- 看護師は，これらをだいたい理解して，高齢者の家族にアドヴァイスできることが望まれる．

WORD LIST

訳語は本テキストで使用している意味だけを示した．

A

abdominal pain　疝痛　61
abnormal sensation　知覚異常　67
abortion　妊娠中絶，流産　43
absorbent pad　尿とりパッド　95
acupuncturist　鍼灸師　5
acute nephritis　急性腎炎　23
aging　加齢　89
agitation　興奮　95
airway obstruction　気道閉塞　53
alcohol abuse　アルコール乱用　33
allergic rhinitis　アレルギー性鼻炎　37
ambulance attendant　救急隊員　53
analgesic　鎮痛薬　73
aneurysm　動脈瘤　67
angina　狭心症　59
anorexia　拒食症　33
anticoagulant　抗凝血薬　67
anus　肛門　21
anxiety　不安症　33
aphasia　失語症　67
appendix　盲腸　21
appointment slip　予約票　17
arrhythmia　不整脈　59
artery　動脈　69
arthritis　関節炎　25
artificial respiration　人工呼吸　53
aspiration　呼吸，吸引，誤嚥　87
assessment　アセスメント，審査，判定　91
astigmatism　乱視　35
asymptomatic　無症状　55
atrium　心房　69

B

balanced diet　バランスの取れた食事　99
bandage　包帯　79
barrier-free　バリアフリー　97
bath treatment　入浴療法　39
bathroom　トイレ　63
bed control　ベッドコントロール　65
bed light　ウォールライト　65
bedpan　便器　9
bedrail　ベッド柵　101
bedrest　床上安静　79
bedridden　寝たきり　101
bedside table　床頭台　65
bed-wetting　夜尿症　31
benign tumor　良性腫瘍　57
bile　胆汁　27
bill　請求書　17
biofeedback　バイオフィードバック（BF）法　69
birth control　避妊　43
bisphosphonates　ビスフォスフォネート製剤　89
bladder　膀胱　41
bleeding　出血　49
blood pressure gauge　血圧計　7
blood sugar level　血糖値　75
blood test　血液検査　75
bloody sputum　血痰　87
bloody stools　血便　61
bowel sounds　腸音　29
brain tumor　脳腫瘍　45
breath odor　口臭　49
bridge　ブリッジ　47
bronchitis　気管支炎　31
bulimia　過食症　33

C

calcium　カルシウム　89
calculus　結石　27
call bell　呼出ベル　65
cane　ステッキ　97
cardiac arrest　心停止　53
cardiac catheterization　心カテーテル検査　59

103

cardiac massage　心臓マッサージ　53
caregiver　介護者　91
care manager　ケアマネジャー　91
care recipient　要介護者　91
carrier　保菌者　85
cashier　会計窓口　17
cavity　虫歯　47
cesarean section　帝王切開　83
chapped skin　ひび割れの生じた肌　39
chart　カルテ　15
chemotherapy　化学療法　57
chest pain　胸痛，胸が苦しい状態　11, 59
chickenpox　水疱瘡　31
(chronic)bronchitis　(慢性)気管支炎　19
cholangiogram　胆管造影　27
clot　血栓，凝血　67
cold　風邪，感冒　19
colic　疝痛　61
collapsed lung　気胸　55
colon cancer　大腸癌　21
colostomy　人工肛門　71
commode　ポータブルトイレ　95
complete blood count (CBC)　全血球計算，全血算　51
complication　合併症　99
congestive heart failure　うっ血性心不全　59
constipation　便秘　61
consultation card　診察カード　15
contraception　避妊　43
convulsion(s)　痙攣，ひきつけ　31
cough　咳　87
counseling　カウンセリング　99
cracked skin　ひび割れの生じた肌　39
crash cart　緊急用(医療処置)カート　51
crown　歯冠　47
CT (computed tomography)　コンピュータ断層撮影装置　55
cyanosis　チアノーゼ　53
cystitis　膀胱炎　23

D

dairy products　乳製品　89
dayroom　デイルーム　97
decayed tooth　虫歯　47
decubitus ulcer　褥瘡，床ずれ　93
deep breathing　深呼吸　71
defibrillation　細動除去　53
deformity　変形　25
dehydration　脱水状態　11
delivery　出産　43
delivery room　分娩室　83
dental caries　虫歯　47
dental hygienist　歯科衛生士　49
dental implant　歯のインプラント　49
dentist　歯科医師　3
denture　義歯・入れ歯　47
depression　うつ　33
dermatology　皮膚科　15
desiccated skin　かさかさの肌　39
diabetic coma　糖尿病性昏睡　75
diabetic retinopathy　糖尿病性網膜症　75
diaper rash　おむつかぶれ　31
diarrhea　下痢　61
dietitian　栄養士　5
differential diagnosis　鑑別診断　27
difficulty breathing　呼吸困難　55
digitalis　ジギタリス　69
diphtheria　ジフテリア　31
discharge　分泌物，排出物，退院　37
dizziness　めまい　11
doctor　医師　3
drain　ドレーン　55
drainage　排膿　49
dressing　包帯　79
dressing change　包帯や帯具の交換　71
drip infusion kit　点滴装置　7
drug addiction　薬物中毒　33
dry skin　かさかさの肌　39
duodenum　十二指腸　21, 73
dysarthria　構音障害　67
dyspnea　呼吸困難　55

E

earache 耳痛 37
eardrum 鼓膜 37
eczema 湿疹 39
edema 浮腫 23
elderly person 高齢者 91
electrocardiogram 心電図 7
elevated temperature 発熱 11
embolus 栓子 67
emesis 嘔吐 13
encephalitis 脳炎 31
endoscope 内視鏡 7
enlargement 腫脹 25
ENT (ear, nose and throat) 耳鼻科 15
episiotomy 会陰切開 83
erosion ただれ 39
erythema 紅斑 39
erythrocyte 赤血球 27
esophageal reflux 食道狭窄 21
esophagus 食道 21, 73
exophthalmia 眼球突出症 81

F

fainting 失神 13
farsightedness 遠視 35
fatigue 疲労 85
feeding tube 栄養管 73
fetus 胎児 43
fever 発熱 11
filling 充填 47
Foley catheter フォーリー・カテーテル 41
follow-up 再調査 77
food cart 配膳車 63
forced fluids 強制輸液 23
four-bed ward 四人部屋 63

G

gallbladder 胆嚢 27
gastritis 胃炎 21

German measles 風疹 31
glaucoma 緑内障 35
goiter 甲状腺 81
gown ガウン 9
guide dog 盲導犬 99
gum recession 歯肉切除(術) 49

H

halitosis 口臭 49
hard of hearing 難聴 99
have a skin irritation 皮膚がかぶれる 39
hay fever 花粉症 37
headache 頭痛 13
hearing aid 補聴器 99
heart attack 心臓発作 59
heart murmur 心雑音 59
heat rash あせも 31
hemoptysis 喀血 87
hemorrhoids 痔 61
hives じんま疹 13, 39
hoarseness 嗄声 81
home care 在宅ケア 93
home helper ホームヘルパー 95
home renovation 住宅改修 91
hormone replacement therapy (HRT) ホルモン療法 89
house call 往診 93
hygiene 衛生 101
hyperthyroidism 甲状腺機能亢進症 81
hypoglycemia 低血糖 75

I

ice pillow 氷枕 87
impaired circulation 循環障害 79
incision 切開 71
incontinence 失禁 95
independence 自立 97
induced labor 誘発分娩 83
inflamed skin 炎症を起こした肌 39

inflammation　炎症　25
influenza　インフルエンザ　19
injection　注射　75
insomnia　不眠(症)　93
insulin shock　インスリン・ショック　75
insurance card　保険証　15
insurance premiums　保険料　77
internal medicine　内科　15
interphone　インターフォン　65
intestinal obstruction　腸閉塞　61
intestines　腸　73
intraocular lens　眼内レンズ　35
intubation　挿管　73
ISG(immune serum globulin)　免疫血清グロブリン　85
isolation　隔離　85
itching　かゆみ，掻痒症　39

J

jaundice　黄疸　85

K

keloid　ケロイド　71
kidney　腎臓　23
kidney transplant　腎移植　23

L

lack of exercise　運動不足　75
Lamaze method　ラマーズ法　43
large intestine　大腸　21
laser treatment　レーザー治療　35
lesion　傷　71
leukocyte　白血球　27
leukopenia　白血球減少症　45
level of consciousness　意識レベル　101
lifesaving equipment　緊急用(医療処置)カート　51
liquid diet　流動食　29
liquid food　流動食　73
list of charges　請求書　17

local anesthesia　局所麻酔　43
long-term care insurance　介護保険　91
loss of sensation　感覚喪失　29
low birth weight infant　低出生体重児　83
lumbar anesthesia　腰椎麻酔　29
lumpectomy　乳腺腫瘤摘出　57
lymph gland　リンパ腺　57

M

macular degeneration　黄斑変性　35
malignant tumor　悪性腫瘍　57
malnutrition　低栄養　101
mammography　マンモグラフィー　57
mastectomy　乳房切除　57
measles　はしか　31
medical engineer　メディカルエンジニア　5
medical history form　問診票　15
medical office worker　医療事務員　3
medical secretary　医療秘書　3
medical technologist　臨床検査技師　5
menstruation　生理　43
metabolic rate　代謝率　81
metastasis　転移　57
midwife　助産師　83
molar　大臼歯　47
morning sickness　つわり　43
morning stiffness　朝のこわばり　25
MRI(magnetic resonance imaging)　核磁気共鳴映像装置　55
mumps　おたふくかぜ　31

N

nasal cannula　経鼻カニューレ　93
national health insurance　国民健康保険　15
nausea　吐き気　29
nearsightedness　近視　35
needle biopsy and cytodiagnosis　穿刺吸引細胞診　57
neurology　神経科　15
neurosis　神経症　33

nosebleed　鼻出血　37
number ticket　番号札　15
nurse　看護師　3
nurses' station　看護ステーション　63

O

obesity　肥満　75
obstetrician　産科医　83
obstetrics and gynecology (OB-Gyn)　産婦人科　15
occlusion　閉塞　67
occupational therapist　作業療法士　5
oily skin　脂性の肌　39
ointment　軟膏　39
ophthalmology　眼科　15
orthopedic surgery　整形外科手術　79
orthopedics　整形外科　15
osteoarthritis　変形性関節症　25
outpatient (counter)　外来(窓口)　77
overweight　肥満　75
oximeter　パルスオキシメーター　53
oxygen　酸素　53
oxygen concentrator　酸素濃縮器　93
oxygen mask　酸素マスク　93

P

painkiller　鎮痛薬　73
paleness　顔面蒼白　11
pallor　顔面蒼白　11
papules　丘疹　39
paralysis　麻痺　67
paramedic　救急救命士　51
parenteral nutrition　腸管外栄養　73
parking lot ticket　駐車チケット　17
partially deaf　難聴　99
passing gas　おならをすること　13
patient card　診察カード　15
pediatrics　小児科　15
period　月経　43
perspiration　発汗　11

pertussis　百日咳　31
PET (positron emission tomography) scan　PETスキャン　45
pharmacist　薬剤師　5
physical therapist　理学療法士　5
physical therapy　物理(理学)療法　67
physician　医師　3
pimply skin　吹き出物だらけの肌　39
pleurisy　胸膜炎　87
pneumococcus　肺炎球菌　87
pneumonia　肺炎　19
pneumothorax　気胸　55
polyp　ポリープ　61
portable toilet　ポータブルトイレ，ポータブル便器　9, 95
premature birth　早産　83
prescription　処方箋　17
pressure sore　褥瘡，床ずれ　93
private room　個室　63
prostatectomy　前立腺切除術　41
prosthesis　プロテーゼ　57
protective pants　おむつ　95
pruritus　かゆみ，掻痒症　39
psychiatry　精神科　15
public health nurse　保健師　77
puffiness　腫脹，むくみ　39
pulmonary edema　肺水腫　87
pulse ox　パルスオキシメーター　53
pus　膿　79

R

radiation burns　放射線熱傷　45
radioactive iodine　放射性ヨウ素　81
rash　発疹　13
receipt　領収書　17
rectal cancer　直腸癌　21
rectum　直腸　21
recurrence　再発　55
red blood cell　赤血球　27
redness　紅斑　39
referral letter　紹介状　77

referred pain　関連痛　29
regurgitation　逆流　69
rehabilitation　リハビリ　99
relapse　再発　55
remission　緩解　55
renal transplant　腎移植　23
reservation　予約　63
respiratory arrest　呼吸停止　53
restlessness　情動不安　95
restraints　抑制，拘束　101
resuscitation　蘇生　51
retinal detachment　網膜剥離　35
ringing in the ears　耳鳴　11
root canal　根管　47
rubella　風疹　31
rupture　破裂　29

S

salt restriction　塩分制限　59
salve　軟膏　39
sanitation　衛生施設　101
scar　傷痕　71
scarred skin　瘢痕（傷跡）肌　39
sedation　鎮静　61
seeing eye dog　盲導犬　99
self-reliance　自立　97
senior citizen　高齢者　91
sexual dysfunction　性的機能障害　41
shampoo　シャンプー　9
shop　売店　63
shot　注射　75
shower room　シャワー室　63
shuttle bus　シャトルバス　97
side effects　副作用　45
sigmoid colon　S状結腸　21
sinusitis　副鼻腔炎（蓄膿症）　19
skin care　スキンケア　71
sleeplessness　不眠（症）　93
slurred speech　不明瞭言語　67
small intestine　小腸　21

soap　石鹸　9
sore throat　咽頭痛　19，37
sphygmomanometer　血圧計　7
spinal fractures　脊椎骨折　89
spontaneous fractures　特発性骨折　89
steroids　ステロイド類　39
stoma　ストーマ（人工肛門）　71
stomach　胃　21
stomach ulcer　胃潰瘍　21
stomachache　胃痛　13
stone　結石　27
store　売店　63
stress　ストレス　75
stroke　脳卒中，脳溢血　101
surgery　外科　15
sweat　発汗　11
swelling　腫脹，むくみ　25，39
symptom-free　無症状　55
syncope　失神　13

T

tachycardia　頻脈　81
tartar　歯石　49
television（TV）　テレビ　65
terminal care　ターミナルケア　93
tetanus　破傷風　31
thermometer　体温計　7
throbbing pain　疼痛，ずきずきする痛み　13
thrombus　血栓，凝血　67
thyroid crisis　甲状腺中毒症　81
tinnitus　耳鳴　11
toilet　トイレ　63
tonsillitis　扁桃炎　31
toothache　歯痛　47
towel　タオル　9
tracheostomy　気管形成術　81
traction　牽引　79
transfusion　輸血　51
trauma　外傷　51
triage　トリアージ　51

tube feeding　経管栄養　73
tuberculosis(TB)　肺結核　55
turning　寝返り　93
type A(B, C) hepatitis　A(B,C)型肝炎　85

U

undernourishment　低栄養　101
unit secretary　医療事務員　3
ureteral calculus　尿管結石　41
urinal　尿瓶　9
urinalysis　尿検査　23
urinary frequency　頻尿　41
urinary retention　残尿　41
urine test　尿検査　75
urology　泌尿器科　15

V

vaccine　ワクチン　85
valve　弁　69
van　バン　97
vase　花瓶　65
vein　静脈　69
ventricle　心室　69
vertigo　めまい　11
violence　暴力行為　33
viral infection　ウイルス感染　19
visiting nurse　訪問看護師　77
visitors' room　面会室　63
vitamins　ビタミン　99
vomiting　嘔吐　13, 29

W

walker　歩行器　97
wandering　徘徊　95
washbasin　洗面器　65
waterproof sheet　防水シート　95
weakness　だるい，脱力感　11
weight-bearing exercise　加重負荷運動　89

(electric) wheelchair　(電動)車椅子　97
white blood cell　白血球　27
whooping cough　百日咳　31
wisdom tooth　親知らず　47
wound　傷　71

X

X-ray films　X線フィルム，レントゲン写真　45
X-ray technician　放射線技師　5

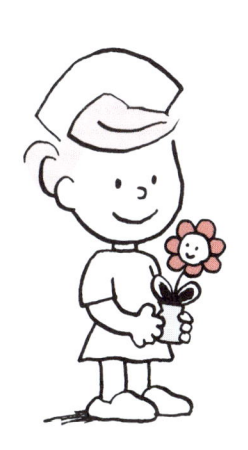